Diabetic Foot
A Comprehensive Guide for Clinicians

Diabetic Foot
A Comprehensive Guide for Clinicians

Editors

Felix Jebasingh K
MBBS MD DM (Endo) DNB (Endo) MNAMS PGDMLE (Med Law)
Associate Professor
Department of Endocrinology, Diabetes and Metabolism
Christian Medical College
Vellore, Tamil Nadu, India

Nihal Thomas
MBBS MD MNAMS DNB (Endo) FRACP (Endo) FRCP (Edin) FRCP (Glasg)
FRCP (Lond) FACP PhD (Copenhagen)
Professor and Head, Unit-1
Department of Endocrinology, Diabetes and Metabolism
Christian Medical College
Vellore, Tamil Nadu, India

Foreword

Andrew JM Boulton

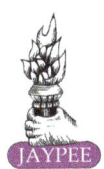

JAYPEE BROTHERS MEDICAL PUBLISHERS
The Health Sciences Publisher
New Delhi | London

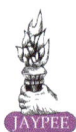 **Jaypee Brothers Medical Publishers (P) Ltd**

Headquarters
EMCA House
23/23-B, Ansari Road, Daryaganj
New Delhi 110 002, India
Landline: +91-11-23272143, +91-11-23272703
+91-11-23282021, +91-11-23245672
E-mail: jaypee@jaypeebrothers.com

Corporate Office
Jaypee Brothers Medical Publishers (P) Ltd.
4838/24, Ansari Road, Daryaganj
New Delhi 110 002, India
Phone: +91-11-43574357
Fax: +91-11-43574314
E-mail: jaypee@jaypeebrothers.com

Overseas Office
JP Medical Ltd.
83, Victoria Street, London
SW1H 0HW (UK)
Phone: +44-20 3170 8910
Fax: +44(0)20 3008 6180
E-mail: info@jpmedpub.com

Website: www.jaypeebrothers.com
Website: www.jaypeedigital.com

© 2023, Jaypee Brothers Medical Publishers

The views and opinions expressed in this book are solely those of the original contributor(s)/author(s) and do not necessarily represent those of editor(s) or publisher of the book.

All rights reserved by the author. No part of this publication may be reproduced, stored or transmitted in any form or by any means, electronic, mechanical, photocopying, recording or otherwise, without the prior permission in writing of the publishers.

All brand names and product names used in this book are trade names, service marks, trademarks or registered trademarks of their respective owners. The publisher is not associated with any product or vendor mentioned in this book.

Medical knowledge and practice change constantly. This book is designed to provide accurate, authoritative information about the subject matter in question. However, readers are advised to check the most current information available on procedures included and check information from the manufacturer of each product to be administered, to verify the recommended dose, formula, method and duration of administration, adverse effects and contraindications. It is the responsibility of the practitioner to take all appropriate safety precautions. Neither the publisher nor the author(s)/editor(s) assume any liability for any injury and/or damage to persons or property arising from or related to use of material in this book.

This book is sold on the understanding that the publisher is not engaged in providing professional medical services. If such advice or services are required, the services of a competent medical professional should be sought.

Every effort has been made where necessary to contact holders of copyright to obtain permission to reproduce copyright material. If any have been inadvertently overlooked, the publisher will be pleased to make the necessary arrangements at the first opportunity. The **CD/DVD-ROM** (if any) provided in the sealed envelope with this book is complimentary and free of cost. **It is Not meant for sale**.

Inquiries for bulk sales may be solicited at: jaypee@jaypeebrothers.com

Diabetic Foot: A Comprehensive Guide for Clinicians / Felix Jebasingh K, Nihal Thomas

First Edition: **2023**

ISBN: 978-93-5465-545-6

DEDICATION

To our special friend and colleague, the late Professor (Dr) Sunil Agarwal, who supported us immensely, as far back as the year 2009. He endorsed us during the formation of the integrated diabetes foot clinic at CMC Vellore, from its initial days.

CONTRIBUTORS

Editors

Felix Jebasingh K MBBS MD DM (Endo) DNB (Endo) MNAMS PGDMLE (Med Law)
Associate Professor
Department of Endocrinology, Diabetes and Metabolism
Christian Medical College
Vellore, Tamil Nadu, India

Nihal Thomas MBBS MD MNAMS DNB (Endo) FRACP (Endo) FRCP (Edin) FRCP (Glasg) FRCP (Lond) FACP PhD (Copenhagen)
Professor and Head, Unit-1
Department of Endocrinology, Diabetes and Metabolism
Christian Medical College
Vellore, Tamil Nadu, India

Associate Editors

Bobeena Rachel Chandy MBBS MD (PMR) DNB
Professor
Department of Physical Medicine and Rehabilitation
Christian Medical College
Vellore, Tamil Nadu, India

Pranay Gaikwad DNB MNAMS DMAS FMAS
Professor and Head, Unit-1
Department of Surgery: General Head and Neck Surgery
Christian Medical College
Vellore, Tamil Nadu, India

Anand John Samuel G BE (Mech) M Phil (HHSM) MBA (HSM)
Superintendenting Engineer, Prosthetic and Orthotic Services
Department of Physical Medicine and Rehabilitation
Christian Medical College
Vellore, Tamil Nadu, India

Kripa Elizabeth Cherian MBBS MD DM (Endo) DNB (Endo)
Associate Professor, Department of Endocrinology, Diabetes and Metabolism
Christian Medical College
Vellore, Tamil Nadu, India

Bharathi K BSc (N)
Charge Nurse and Diabetes Educator
Department of Endocrinology, Diabetes and Metabolism, Christian Medical College
Vellore, Tamil Nadu, India

Flory Christina I BSc (N)
Charge Nurse and Diabetes Educator
Department of Endocrinology, Diabetes and Metabolism, Christian Medical College
Vellore, Tamil Nadu, India

Mathews Edatharayil Kurian MBBS
Research Officer, Department of Endocrinology, Diabetes and Metabolism
Christian Medical College
Vellore, Tamil Nadu, India

Contributors

Contributing Authors

Albert Abhinay Kota MBBS MS DNB MRCS MCh
Associate Professor
Department of Vascular Surgery
Christian Medical College
Vellore, Tamil Nadu, India

Anand John Samuel G BE (Mech) M Phil (Hospital and Health System Management) MBA (Health Services Management)
Superintendenting Engineer, Prosthetic and Orthotic Services
Department of Physical Medicine and Rehabilitation
Christian Medical College
Vellore, Tamil Nadu, India

Bharathi K BSc (N)
Charge Nurse and Diabetes Educator
Department of Endocrinology, Diabetes and Metabolism
Christian Medical College
Vellore, Tamil Nadu, India

Bobeena Rachel Chandy MBBS MD (PMR) DNB
Professor
Department of Physical Medicine and Rehabilitation
Christian Medical College
Vellore, Tamil Nadu, India

B Vinod Jacob DPO ISPO Cat II
Prosthetist and Orthotist
Department of Physical Medicine and Rehabilitation
Christian Medical College
Vellore, Tamil Nadu, India

Ezhilarasi V BSc (N)
Diabetes Educator
Department of Endocrinology, Diabetes and Metabolism
Christian Medical College
Vellore, Tamil Nadu, India

Felix Jebasingh K MBBS MD DM (Endo) DNB (Endo) MNAMS PGDMLE (Med Law)
Associate Professor
Department of Endocrinology, Diabetes and Metabolism
Christian Medical College
Vellore, Tamil Nadu, India

Flory Christina I BSc (N)
Charge Nurse and Diabetes Educator
Department of Endocrinology, Diabetes and Metabolism
Christian Medical College
Vellore, Tamil Nadu, India

Gourav Sannyasi MBBS MD (PMR)
Senior Resident, Department of Physical Medicine and Rehabilitation
Christian Medical College
Vellore, Tamil Nadu, India

Ida Nirmal BSc (N) MSc (N) ET (Enterostomal Therapist)
Professor and Nurse Manager
Colorectal Unit, College of Nursing
Christian Medical College
Vellore, Tamil Nadu, India

Ilakkiya J RN
Diabetes Educator, Department of Endocrinology, Diabetes and Metabolism
Christian Medical College
Vellore, Tamil Nadu, India

Jinson Paul MBBS MD DM (Endo)
Assistant Professor
Department of Endocrinology, Diabetes and Metabolism
Christian Medical College
Vellore, Tamil Nadu, India

Johns T Johnson MBBS MD (Gen Med)
Senior Resident, Department of Endocrinology, Diabetes and Metabolism
Christian Medical College
Vellore, Tamil Nadu, India

Contributors

Kelita George MBBS Postgraduate Fellowship in Diabetes
PG Resident
Department of Endocrinology, Diabetes and Metabolism
Christian Medical College
Vellore, Tamil Nadu, India

Kripa Elizabeth Cherian MBBS MD DM (Endo) DNB (Endo)
Associate Professor
Department of Endocrinology, Diabetes and Metabolism
Christian Medical College
Vellore, Tamil Nadu, India

Naveen Cherian Thomas MBBS MD (PMR)
Assistant Professor
Department of Physical Medicine and Rehabilitation
Christian Medical College
Vellore, Tamil Nadu, India

Nihal Thomas MBBS MD MNAMS DNB (Endo) FRACP (Endo) FRCP (Edin) FRCP (Glasg) FRCP (Lond) FACP PhD (Copenhagen)
Professor and Head, Unit-1
Department of Endocrinology, Diabetes and Metabolism
Christian Medical College
Vellore, Tamil Nadu, India

Pranay Gaikwad DNB MNAMS DMAS FMAS
Professor and Head, Unit-1
Department of Surgery: General Head and Neck Surgery
Christian Medical College
Vellore, Tamil Nadu, India

Ruth Volena D BSc (N)
Diabetes Educator
Department of Endocrinology, Diabetes and Metabolism
Christian Medical College
Vellore, Tamil Nadu, India

Sandeep Kumar Agarwal MBBS MD DM (Endo)
Assistant Professor
Department of Endocrinology, Diabetes and Metabolism
Christian Medical College
Vellore, Tamil Nadu, India

Shirly Jennifer N BSc (N)
Diabetes Educator
Department of Endocrinology, Diabetes and Metabolism
Christian Medical College
Vellore, Tamil Nadu, India

Shivendra Verma MBBS MD DM (Endo)
Senior Resident
Department of Endocrinology, Diabetes and Metabolism
Christian Medical College
Vellore, Tamil Nadu, India

Sunil Agarwal (Late) MBBS MS
Former Professor and Head
Department of Vascular Surgery
Christian Medical College
Vellore, Tamil Nadu, India

Sunitha R BSc (N)
Diabetes Educator
Department of Endocrinology, Diabetes and Metabolism
Christian Medical College
Vellore, Tamil Nadu, India

Vasanth Mark Samuel MBBS MS MRCS
Associate Professor, Unit-1
Department of Surgery
Christian Medical College
Vellore, Tamil Nadu, India

Venkata Sandeep MBBS MD (Gen Med)
Senior Resident
Department of Endocrinology, Diabetes and Metabolism
Christian Medical College
Vellore, Tamil Nadu, India

Vennela Devarapalli MBBS MD (Gen Med)
PDF (Diabetology)
PG Resident
Department of Endocrinology, Diabetes and Metabolism
Christian Medical College
Vellore, Tamil Nadu, India

FOREWORD

It is a pleasure and honor for me to write the foreword to this excellent book edited by Felix Jebasingh and Nihal Thomas from the Department of Endocrinology, Diabetes and Metabolism at the Christian Medical College, Vellore, Tamil Nadu, India. I cannot think of a more appropriate setting for all the authors who have contributed to this most interesting and up-to-date book, which should be standard reading for those with an interest in looking after people with diabetes. This very practical book is beautifully illustrated, and interspersed between the chapters, one finds the short biographies of leaders in the field of the diabetic foot from India and worldwide; some of those giants in the area of diabetic foot care are from India, and are still working despite being retired. Those from overseas are physicians and surgeons who have contributed so much to our understanding of the pathogenesis, management, and indeed prevention of diabetic foot problems. Most notable amongst these are Jean-Martin Charcot, after whom the neuroarthropathy seen in diabetic patients with neuropathy was first described, and Paul Brand, the surgeon who was born in the hills to the west of Madras (now Chennai) and who worked for many years at CMC Vellore, and it was Brand who instructed us in the management of the neuropathic foot in both leprosy and diabetes. Many young physicians reading this book may not be aware of the major contribution that Brand made to the treatment of the insensitive foot but he will be best remembered for his quotation that "pain is God's greatest gift to mankind" and for promoting the use of total contact casts in the management of neuropathic foot ulcers.

The editors have gathered a team of true experts in this area and I recommend this book to anybody with an interest in the diagnosis, management, surgical treatment, and indeed prevention of diabetic foot ulcers. Included in this book in a logical order are the anatomy and biomechanics of the foot followed by chapters on causal pathways, neuropathy, peripheral arterial disease, and then infections of the diabetic foot. Finally, there are chapters on routine podiatric care and other therapies including surgery. I am particularly happy to see that the editors have seen it appropriate to include a final chapter on "Recent advances in diabetic foot management." In modern medicine, any textbook is rapidly out of date in terms of recent developments. The editors of this book have appropriately tried to update this book with last minute developments.

I am sure that all those who read it will benefit greatly from this text and I again thank Jebasingh and Thomas for gathering together such an expert team.

Andrew JM Boulton MD DSc FICP FRCP FACP
Professor of Medicine, University of Manchester,
Division of Diabetes, Endocrinology and Gastroenterology
Consultant Physician, Manchester Royal Infirmary, Manchester, United Kingdom
Visiting Professor of Medicine, University of Miami, Miami, Florida, USA
President, International Diabetes Federation
Past-President, European Association for the Study of Diabetes

PREFACE

Disease of the foot resulting from diabetes is an often serious, yet overlooked complication. The burden of uncontrolled diabetes, causing peripheral neuropathy and diabetes foot in India, is alarming. This book aims to provide a comprehensive overview of the foot in diabetes, its management, and would not have been possible without the collective efforts of our team.

The legacy of Paul Brand who initiated the work in 1948 in handling the foot in leprosy has left us with a lamp that lights the way for the management of the foot in diabetes. Dr Ashish Macaden and his colleagues, from the department of physical medicine and rehabilitation, provided immense support in setting up a foundation and helped us to develop a conceptual framework for the integrated diabetes foot clinic.

Dr Felix who spearheads the integrated diabetes foot clinic and whose ideation led to the fruition of this book, his brainchild. Mr Anand Samuel of the department of prosthetics and orthotics led a world class unit to work hand in glove to generate high quality prosthetics without hesitation, all while maintaining a high output. Dr Mathews helped rejuvenate this manuscript through its various phases and created poetry with a prosaic background, on the diabetes foot. Professor Suranjan Bhattacharjee, with his enlightening presence and ability to think out of the box under the most intriguing circumstances, was instrumental in expanding the scope of our work to the CMC Vellore, Chittoor campus. Our Diabetes Educators, whose competence has gone beyond imaginable boundaries, have raised the bar way ahead of the quantum of natural excellence; their presence and contribution to the system penetrate the normal perceptions of imagination.

We hope that our creation adds significantly to your practice in the field, and provides you with the same sense of fulfillment we achieved, in writing it.

Nihal Thomas

ACKNOWLEDGMENTS

The multidisciplinary overlap between several clinical and nonclinical units is a strong feature of endocrinology. This book would not have been possible but for the strong academic links that the Department of Endocrinology shares with several other departments at CMC Vellore. The enthusiasm and dedication of all our colleagues in the departments of vascular surgery, general surgery, and physical medicine and rehabilitation, prosthetics and orthotics in keeping the ship steady over the years and helping in deciphering complex clinical problems as a team. The care for patients is foundational for such a significant output.

We would like to thank M/s Jaypee Brothers Medical Publishers (P) Ltd, New Delhi, India, especially grateful to Shri Jitendar P Vij (Group Chairman), Mr Ankit Vij (Managing Director), Mr MS Mani (Group President), and also a note of thanks to Dr Richa Saxena (Associate Director, Professional Publishing), Ms Himani Pandey (Development Editor), Ms Seema Dogra (Cover Visualizer) and the entire Production Team at Jaypee Brothers, for managing this project well.

Felix Jebasingh K
Nihal Thomas

CONTENTS

CHAPTER 1: Introduction to Diabetic Foot Care — 1
Sandeep Kumar Agarwal, Bharathi K, Vasanth Mark Samuel, Felix Jebasingh K, Nihal Thomas

CHAPTER 2: Anatomy and Biomechanics of the Diabetic Foot — 8
Bobeena Rachel Chandy, Gourav Sannyasi

CHAPTER 3: Peripheral Neuropathy: Clinical Approach — 23
Jinson Paul, Shivendra Verma, Kripa Elizabeth Cherian, Flory Christina I, B Vinod Jacob, Felix Jebasingh K, Nihal Thomas

CHAPTER 4: Diabetic Foot Ulcers: Clinical Approach — 43
Jinson Paul, Felix Jebasingh K, Kripa Elizabeth Cherian, Anand John Samuel G, Ruth Volena D, Nihal Thomas

CHAPTER 5: The Charcot Foot: Clinical Features and Management — 65
Venkata Sandeep, Ilakkiya J, Bharathi K, Anand John Samuel G, Felix Jebasingh K, Nihal Thomas

CHAPTER 6: Osteomyelitis of the Diabetic Foot — 89
Kelita George, Johns T Johnson, Kripa Elizabeth Cherian, Shirly Jennifer N, Felix Jebasingh K, Nihal Thomas

CHAPTER 7: Peripheral Vascular Disease: Clinical Approach — 103
Albert Abhinay Kota, Sunil Agarwal (Late)

CHAPTER 8: Footwear and Offloading Aids in Diabetic Foot — 117
Bobeena Rachel Chandy, Naveen Cherian Thomas

CHAPTER 9: Callus Removal, Debridement and Foot Care — 134
Bharathi K, Flory Christina I, Ruth Volena D, Shirly Jennifer N, Ezhilarasi V, Sunitha R, Ilakkiya J, Vennela Devarapalli, Felix Jebasingh K, Nihal Thomas

CHAPTER 10: Negative Pressure Wound Therapy — 149
Ida Nirmal, Albert Abhinay Kota, Bharathi K, Felix Jebasingh K

Contents

CHAPTER 11: Surgery of the Diabetic Foot   **159**
Pranay Gaikwad

CHAPTER 12: Necrotizing Fasciitis in Diabetes   **168**
Pranay Gaikwad

CHAPTER 13: Recent Advances in Diabetic Foot Management   **179**
Sandeep Kumar Agarwal, Felix Jebasingh K, Nihal Thomas

Index   **185**

CHAPTER 1

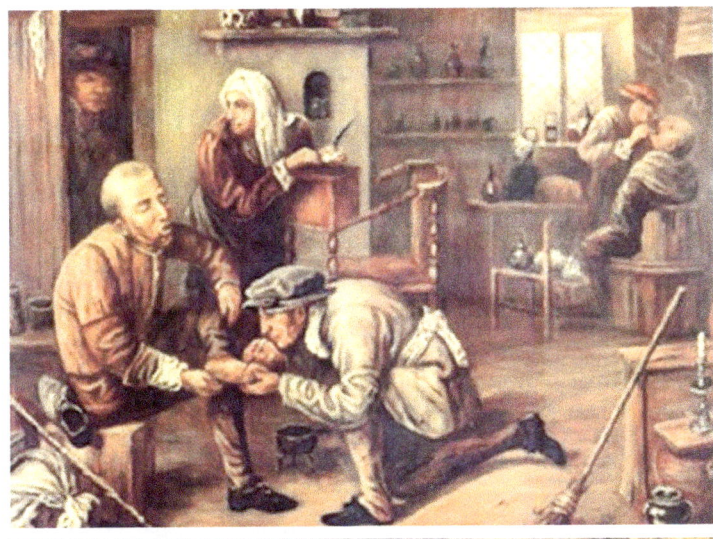

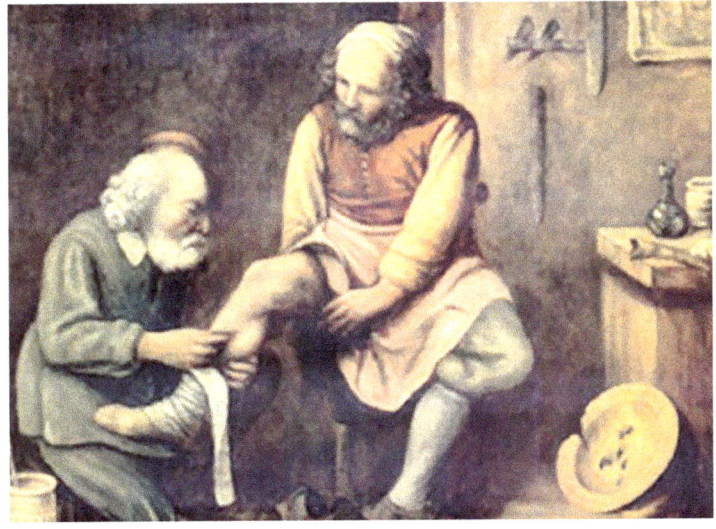

"The foot is a masterpiece of engineering and a work of art".
—***Leonardo da Vinci***

Introduction to Diabetic Foot Care

Sandeep Kumar Agarwal, Bharathi K, Vasanth Mark Samuel,
Felix Jebasingh K, Nihal Thomas

INTRODUCTION

Diabetes mellitus is a group of metabolic diseases characterized by hyperglycemia resulting from defects in insulin secretion, insulin action, or both. It is well known that diabetes may lead to a number of micro- and macrovascular complications which include peripheral neuropathy, peripheral vascular disease, increased risk of foot infection and delayed wound healing.[1]

Out of all the complications, diabetic foot disease (DFD) can be considered as one of the most devastating and demoralizing complications of diabetes. The Diabetic foot is defined as a group of disorders wherein neuropathy, ischemia or infection may lead to tissue breakdown and a potential to progress toward amputation. The lifetime risk for the development of a diabetic foot ulcer (DFU) in patients with diabetes may range from 15 to 25%, and this is known to precede amputation in 85% of cases.[2,3] The rate of lower limb amputation in patients with DM is 15 times higher than in patients without diabetes and approximately 50–70% of all lower limb amputations are due to DFU.[4] Every 20 seconds a lower limb is lost due to diabetes and it is the most common cause of non-traumatic lower limb amputation.[5] It may severely impair the quality of life of patients by affecting productivity, social participation, and livelihood. These amputations also precipitate an increase in mortality rate. However, there are a number of preventable causes for amputation particularly in low socioeconmic societies, such as a lack of sanitation and hygiene, socio-cultural practices such as barefoot walking inside the house and at religious places, lack of awareness on the use of proper footwear and a dearth of foot care clinics which may add to the burden of foot disease related to diabetes mellitus.

DFD includes several pathologies, particularly diabetic peripheral neuropathy (DPN), peripheral arterial disease (PAD), and infections (**Flowchart 1**). DPN results in sensory, motor and autonomic nerve dysfunction leading to DFU. When screening, almost all patients with diabetes who are undergoing foot-related surgical procedures, a majority are found to have neuropathy.[6]

Introduction to Diabetic Foot Care

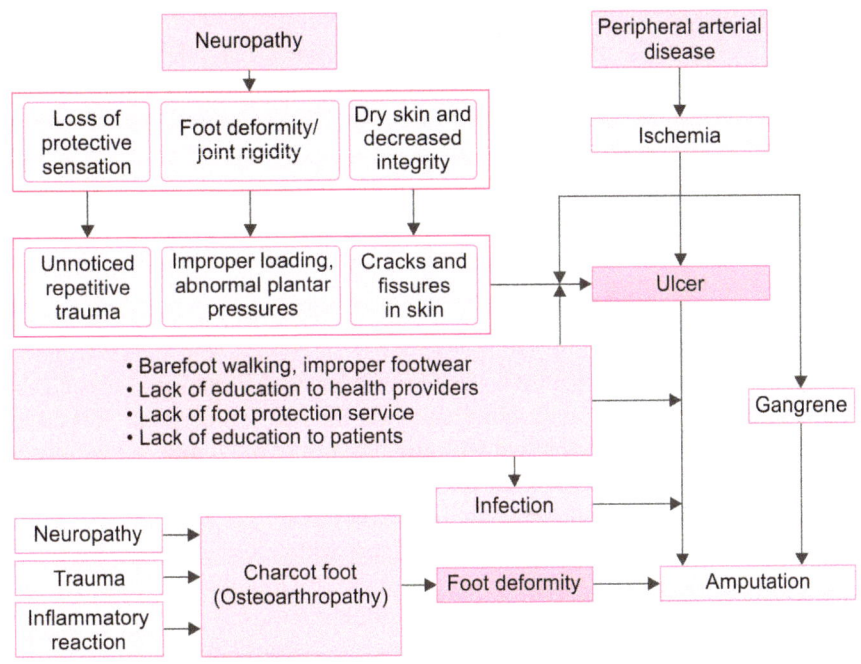

FLOWCHART 1: Risk factors and mechanism for foot ulcer and amputation.

Peripheral neuropathy is associated with high rates of skin breakdown and neuropathic fractures due to the inability to perceive pain sensation. The inciting trauma may include ill-fitting shoes or minor sprains and strains. Without protective sensation, a patient with peripheral neuropathy lacks the physical symptoms that would alert healthy individuals to examine their feet, thereby increasing the extent of skin damage, prior to their presentation for treatment. Patients with moderate to severe sensory loss are shown to have a seven-time higher risk of developing a first DFU when compared to patients with preserved sensation.[7]

Autonomic dysfunction, as a result of neuropathy, may also contribute to ulcer formation. It affects both physiologic secretions and the arterio-venous systems leading to dry and fragile skin. This in turn increases the risk of cracks, fissures and skin breakdown, and thereafter, the risk of infection. Motor neuropathy may lead to structural changes to the foot and these changes are partly due to muscular weakness and imbalance caused by intrinsic atrophy manifesting as hammer toes, mallet toe, claw toes, a prominent metatarsal head and other deformities. Such deformities, in turn change pressure patterns on the foot resulting in certain areas becoming more susceptible to trauma or ulceration.

Charcot neuropathic osteoarthropathy (CN) or Charcot foot is also a part of DFD that may affect the bones, joints, and soft tissues of the foot and ankle, characterized by inflammation in its early phase. Diabetes-related Charcot's arthropathy has a reported prevalence between 0.08 and 13%.[8] Patients with diabetic foot are also

Introduction to Diabetic Foot Care

more likely to present with other diabetes-related complications inclusive of nephropathy, retinopathy, ischemic heart disease and cerebrovascular disease which further aggravate DFD. A combination of neuropathy, abnormal load bearing by the foot, repeated microtrauma, and metabolic abnormalities of bone leads to osteolysis, fractures, dislocation and deformities.

Diagnosing DFD involves a need for a thorough foot examination, which aids in the detection of disease at an early stage. Screening for peripheral neuropathy and PAD may help identify patients at risk of foot ulcers. A history of ulcers or amputations and poor glycemic control, increases the risk further. Examination of the feet at each follow-up visit for any active disease such as ulceration or gangrene is extremely crucial. Clinicians should look for lesions such as cracks, skin fissures, deformed nails, fungal infections, macerated web spaces, calluses and deformities such as claw toes, hammer toes and pes cavus which increase the risk of ulceration. It is advisable to assess the temperature of the feet with the dorsum of the hand. A cold foot might suggest ischemia, and increased warmth with redness and swelling might suggest inflammation such as cellulitis or an acute Charcot foot.

Screening should be done to identify patients with a loss of protective sensation (LOPS) in the feet. Most guidelines recommend the 10 g monofilament for neuropathy assessment in people with diabetes. This monofilament exerts a 10 g buckling force when it bends. An inability to sense a 10 g pressure is consistent with LOPS. The test may be combined with another test to screen for neuropathy, such as a biothesiometer or a graduated tuning fork (Rydel Seiffer) to assess the vibration perception threshold.

One should ask for a history of intermittent claudication and rest pain, which may suggest PAD. The ankle brachial index is an easy adjunct bedside measure to diagnose PAD (**Flowchart 2**). It is the ratio of the highest systolic blood pressure at

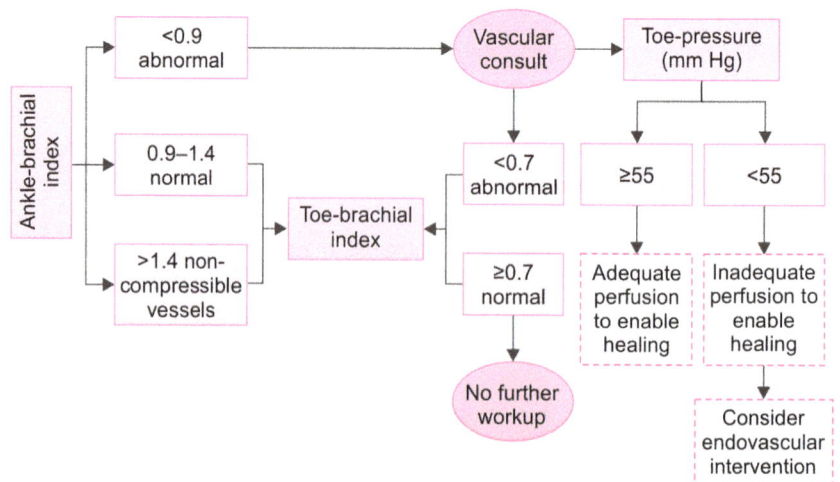

FLOWCHART 2: The evaluation of peripheral artery disease in patients with diabetes.

the ankle (dorsalis pedis artery or posterior tibial artery) to the systolic blood pressure at the arm, and is measured using a Doppler device. People with diabetes can often have falsely raised ankle brachial index levels as a result of poor compressibility from calcified arteries. Availability of equipment, time constraints, and lack of training are also major barriers to ankle brachial index testing in the primary care setting.

Peripheral arterial disease is frequently found with neuropathy, in the diabetic patient and can contribute to foot complications. Approximately 50% of patients with DFD are found to have some degree of PAD. Compared to patients with diabetes and Charcot neuropathy, patients with DFUs are significantly more likely to have PAD, critical limb ischemia and more often require revascularization (**Flowchart 2**). Endothelial damage and vessel sclerosis of both large and small vessels leads to decreased peripheral perfusion. Hence, patients are at an increased risk for ulceration and leads to impaired wound-healing and infection-fighting abilities.

Patients with diabetes have an impaired ability to mount an inflammatory response to infection (immunopathy). Impaired neutrophil function, chemotaxis, phagocytosis, as well as a decreased T-cell response have been found in patients with diabetes versus those without diabetes. Hyperglycemia could be one of the etiological factors behind this, which impairs host defenses at the cellular level, affecting leukocytes, macrophages and other cell types. PAD and immunopathy do not directly cause ulceration; however, these patient factors can increase the risk of diabetic foot complications in those with diabetic neuropathy.

Based on the initial assessment, patients may be categorized as having a low, moderate, or high risk of diabetic foot (**Fig. 1**). Low risk indicates the presence of callosities alone; medium risk: The presence of deformity, LOPS, or PAD; high risk includes a previous history of amputation or ulceration along with the presence of any two of the following: LOPS, PAD, and lesions or deformities.[9]

The suggested frequency for follow-up is based on the level of risk. In the low risk state, an annual foot assessment should be performed as they could progress to a moderate or high risk state. Emphasis should be on daily foot inspection and monitoring glycemic control. Increased frequency of follow-up is advised in patients at moderate or high risk, such as those with a foot deformity or with a diagnosis of peripheral neuropathy or PAD at initial assessment. Repeat testing for neuropathy is not necessary if diagnosed previously. A quick inspection for a breach in skin integrity or ulceration should suffice. Patients with asymptomatic PAD may be followed up in primary care centers and managed as in guidelines for PAD. Patients with calluses and deformed toe nails should be referred to preventive podiatry services for basic nail and skin care, including debridement of calluses. A timely referral to the foot protection services for control of risk factors in patients with diabetes prevents infection, gangrene, amputation, or death and reduces hospital admissions.

Early and good glycemic control is effective in preventing peripheral neuropathy. Optimal blood glucose and glycated hemoglobin (HbA1c) targets should be discussed with patients and monitored as per the standard guidelines for diabetes care to prevent or slow the progression of peripheral neuropathy.

Introduction to Diabetic Foot Care

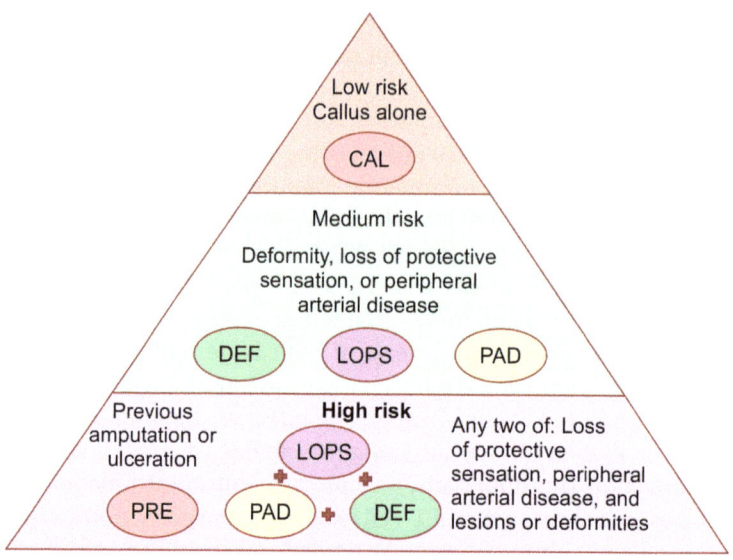

(CAL: callous; DEF: deformity; LOPS: loss of protective sensation; PAD: peripheral arterial disease; PRE: previous amputation)

FIG. 1: Assessment of risk of the diabetic foot.

People with diabetes or their caregivers, or both should be educated on the importance of blood glucose control and modifiable cardiovascular risk factors such as healthy eating habits and lifestyle patterns, regular physical exercise, maintenance of ideal body weight and cessation of smoking and alcohol. While offering modifications in lifestyle, one should consider the patient's cultural as well as religious beliefs and also the social and family support available.

Evidence for the effectiveness of patient education on foot care is lacking. Previously done randomized controlled trials have shown that brief foot care education alone does have a positive influence on patient knowledge and behavior on the short term, but it is ineffective in preventing DFUs. However, education in a structured, organized, and repetitive manner, combined with preventive interventions may prevent foot related problems.

Another less emphasized and ignored aspect of footcare is the usage of appropriate footwear. The sole should be neither too hard nor too soft with a Shore value between 8 and 15 A. Commercially available footwear are often occlusive and causing excessive sweating, thereby precipitating fungal infections, particularly in tropical countries. Bare foot walking is a major risk factor for a succeeding ulcer, especially in patients with neuropathy. Moreover, barefoot walking is rather common amongst people in the many indigenous populations. Patient compliance with regards to the prescribed footwear is usually poor, particularly at home and hence this should be reinforced. Patients with plantar ulcers at the forefoot or heel may be offered offloading footwear to allow ulcer healing and prevent recurrence.

Patients with a life- or limb-threatening problem such as foot ulceration with fever or any signs of sepsis; ulceration with limb ischemia; gangrene, or a suspected deep seated soft tissue or bone infection indicated by either a grossly swollen foot with shiny skin and patches of discoloration or a gritty feel to the bone during a probe to bone test in an open wound should be immediately referred to a specialized diabetic foot center; which are frequently lacking.

Poor outcomes of foot complications in resource poor settings may include the shortage of trained healthcare workers for diabetes care, lack of awareness of footcare among patients and healthcare providers, non-existent podiatry services, shortage of medications and dressing supply, long distances for patients to travel to the clinic, delay by patients in seeking timely medical care or by untrained healthcare providers in referring patients with serious complications for a specialist opinion, lack of the concept of a team approach, absence of training programs for healthcare professionals and finally, a lack of surveillance activities.

Most ulcers may be prevented with appropriate foot care and screening for risk factors for "the foot at risk", for complications. A good understanding of the various predisposing risk factors, would help in both prevention and treatment of this devastating medical condition.

Therefore, this book aims at providing a comprehensive approach toward the management of diabetic foot amongst those with limited health care resources through an integrated foot care program.

REFERENCES

1. Viswanathan V, Thomas N, Tandon N, Asirvatham A, Rajasekar S, Ramachandran A, et al. Profile of diabetic foot complications and its associated complications – A multicentric study from India. J Assoc Physicians India. 2005;53:933-6.
2. Amin N, Doupis J. Diabetic foot disease: From the evaluation of the "foot at risk" to the novel diabetic ulcer treatment modalities. World J Diabetes. 2016;7(7):153-64.
3. Alexiadou K, Doupis J. Management of diabetic foot ulcers. Diabetes Ther. 2012;3(1):4.
4. Yazdanpanah L, Nasiri M, Adarvishi S. Literature review on the management of diabetic foot ulcer. World J Diabetes. 2015;6(1):37-53.
5. Adiewere P, Gillis RB, Imran Jiwani S, Meal A, Shaw I, Adams GG. A systematic review and meta-analysis of patient education in preventing and reducing the incidence or recurrence of adult diabetes foot ulcers (DFU). Heliyon. 2018;4(5):e00614.
6. Suder, NC, Wukich, DK. Prevalence of diabetic neuropathy in patients undergoing foot and ankle surgery. Foot Ankle Spec. 2012;5(2):97-101.
7. Young MJ, Breddy JL, Veves A, Boulton AJ. The prediction of diabetic neuropathic foot ulceration using vibration perception thresholds. A prospective study. Diabetes Care. 1994;17(6):557-60.
8. Frykberg RG, Belczyk R. Epidemiology of the Charcot foot. Clin Podiatr Med Surg. 2008;25(1):17-28.
9. Boulton AJ, Armstrong DG, Albert SF, Frykberg RG, Hellman R, Kirkman MS, et al. Comprehensive foot examination and risk assessment: A report of the task force of the foot care interest group of the American Diabetes Association, with endorsement by the American Association of Clinical Endocrinologists. Diabetes Care. 2008;31(8):1679-85.

CHAPTER 2

MARY VERGHESE

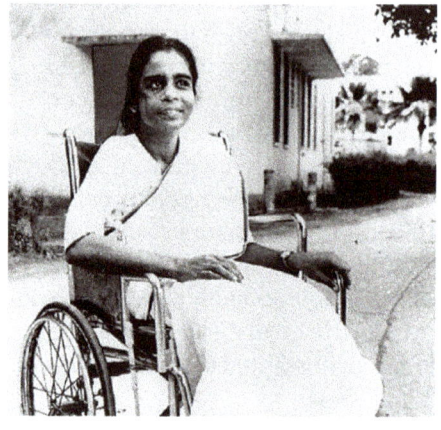

Mary Verghese was born in Kochi, Kerala in South India, on May 26, 1925. She was fiercely independent, and determined to achieve scholarly competence. In the second year of her BA, she decided to become a doctor after being captivated by the story of the medical pioneer, Dr Ida Scudder. She joined the Christian Medical College in Vellore, and graduated in 1952. She aspired to specialize in Gynecology initially, however, the course of her life changed when she had a motor car accident, rendering her paraplegic. Dr Paul Brand saw her potential and advised her to consider an alternative field of medicine, than what she had planned. She trained with him, operating on the hands of leprosy patients, which could be done while seated on a chair. Subsequently, she underwent rehabilitation at the Rehabilitation Center of Royal Perth Hospital in Australia, where she learnt to become independent, and also had a revelation. She came across innovative rehabilitation techniques and recreation for the disabled, which gave her the idea to start a similar department in Vellore. Her dream of establishing a rehabilitation center for those with disabilities was realized when the Rehabilitation Institute at Christian Medical College, Vellore was officially opened in 1966; the first of its kind in India.

Anatomy and Biomechanics of the Diabetic Foot

Bobeena Rachel Chandy, Gourav Sannyasi

INTRODUCTION

"The human foot is a masterpiece of engineering and a work of art" are the words of Leonardo da Vinci, spoken in the 15th century. This is true of the structure and function of an organ that bears the entire weight of the body and has the shock-absorbing capability to endure multiple activities such as walking, running, and jumping. Alterations resulting in the breakdown of architecture and functioning of the foot could lead to major derrangements to the health of an individual.[1]

The diabetic foot is a most serious complication of diabetes mellitus which can result in the loss of a limb. As a result of diabetic peripheral neuropathy, changes that occur in the foot structure affect foot function, subsequently leading to abnormal plantar pressures and eventually ulceration. Prevention of diabetic foot ulceration is possible by early identification of the abnormal biomechanical loading of the insensate foot. Therefore, for this preventive action, it becomes essential to briefly understand the normal biomechanics of the foot and the gait cycle to be able to then identify the changes.[2]

In this chapter, we shall look at the various aspects relating to the anatomy and biomechanics of the foot and the ankle.

ANATOMY

The ankle and foot complex must meet the stability and demands of:
- Providing a stable base of support for the body in a variety of weight-bearing postures without excessive muscular activity and energy expenditure
- Acting as a rigid lever for effective push-off during gait

The stability requirements can be contrasted to the mobility demands of:
- Dampening rotations imposed by the more proximal joints of the lower limbs
- Being flexible enough to absorb the shock of the superimposed body weight as the foot hits the ground
- Permitting the foot to conform to a wide range of changing and varied terrain

Anatomy and Biomechanics of the Diabetic Foot

Bones

Nearly one-fourth of the body's bones are in our feet. The bones of the feet are (**Fig. 1**):
- *Talus*: The bone on top of the foot that forms a joint with the two bones of the lower leg, the tibia and the fibula.
- *Calcaneus*: The largest bone of the foot, which lies beneath the talus to form the heel bone
- *Tarsals*: Five irregularly shaped bones of the midfoot that form the foot's arch
- The tarsal bones are the *cuboid, navicular* and *medial, intermediate*, and *lateral cuneiforms*.
- *Metatarsals*: Five bones (labeled one through five, starting with the big toe) that make up the forefoot.
- *Phalanges (singular: phalanx)*: The 14 bones that make up the toes. The big toe consists of two phalanges—the distal and proximal. The other toes have three.
- *Sesamoids*: Two small pea-shaped bones that lie beneath the head of the first metatarsal in the ball of the foot

To make the understanding of the ankle and foot complex easy, the bones of the foot are divided into three functional segments. These are the *hindfoot* (posterior segment), composed of the talus and calcaneus; the *midfoot* (middle segment), composed of the navicular, cuboid and three cuneiform bones; and the *forefoot* (anterior segment), composed of the metatarsals and the phalanges (**Fig. 2**). These terms are commonly used in descriptions of the normal ankle and foot function and, also foot dysfunction, deformity, or ulcerations.

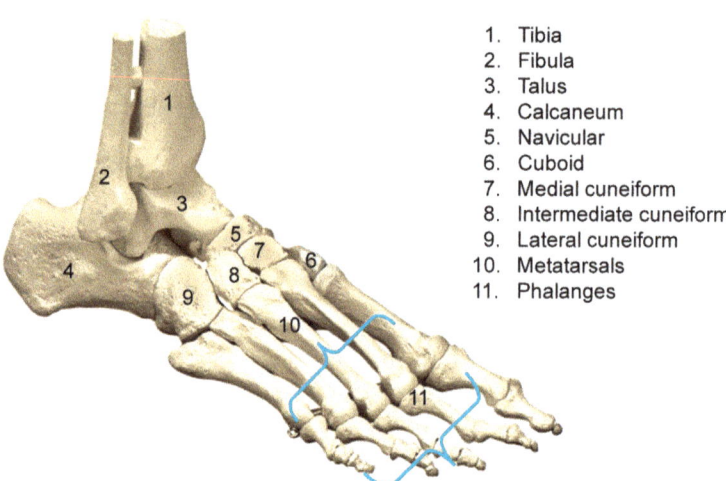

1. Tibia
2. Fibula
3. Talus
4. Calcaneum
5. Navicular
6. Cuboid
7. Medial cuneiform
8. Intermediate cuneiform
9. Lateral cuneiform
10. Metatarsals
11. Phalanges

FIG. 1: Bones of the foot.

Anatomy and Biomechanics of the Diabetic Foot

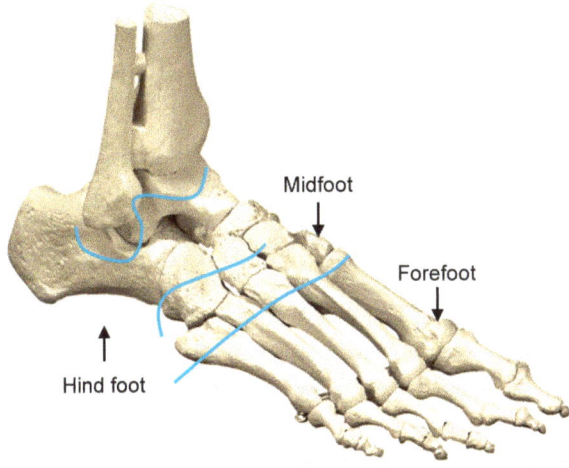

FIG. 2: Functional segments of the foot.

Joints and Articulations

The foot has to act as a pliable platform to support the body weight in the upright posture and as a lever to propel the body forward in walking, running, and jumping. These diverse requirements are met through the integrated movements of its 28 bones that form the 25 component joints.
- *Bones of the lower leg and hind foot*: Tibia, fibula, talus, and calcaneum
- *Joints of the hind foot*: Ankle (tibiotalar) and subtalar
- *Bones of the midfoot*: Cuboid, navicular, and cuneiform (three in numbers)
- *Joints of the midfoot*: Talonavicular, calcaneocuboid, intercuneiform, and tarsometatarsal (TMT)
- *Bones of the forefoot*: Metatarsals (five in numbers), phalanges (14 in numbers), and sesamoid bones (two in numbers)
- *Joints of the forefoot*: Metatarsophalangeal and interphalangeal

Muscles and Tendons

There are four muscles compartments in the lower leg, each separated by fascia. The muscles in these four compartments are collectively referred to as the *extrinsic muscles of the foot* as they originate above the foot, in the leg, and are inserted within the foot.

These are as follows:
- *The superficial posterior compartment*: Gastrocnemius, soleus, and plantaris
- *The deep posterior compartment*: Flexor digitorum longus, flexor hallucis longus, and tibialis posterior. Popliteus is also part of this compartment; however, its insertion is on the tibia

- *The anterior compartment*: Tibialis anterior, extensor hallucis longus, extensor hallucis brevis and peroneus tertius
- *The lateral compartment*: Peroneus longus and peroneus brevis

Muscles within the Foot and the Sole

The internal structure of the sole of the foot is similar to that of the palm. The differences arise from the function of the foot as a supporting structure which has to carry considerable static load while standing and even greater loads at the point of application of severe thrust forces (e.g., push off in running, kicking, landing on the feet, when jumping from height). The sole is divided into skin, superficial fascia, deep fascia, four layers of muscles, and the deep part with the arteries and nerves.

The skin of the sole is thick for protection and firmly adherent to the underlying plantar aponeurosis and crease. These features increase the efficiency of the grip of the sole on the ground. Several smaller muscles deep inside the foot, collectively called the *intrinsic muscles* (because they are contained within the foot), help with toe movements and stabilizing the foot. The extensor hallucis brevis and extensor digitorum brevis are in the dorsum of the foot. They help with extension of the toes. Similarly, flexor hallucis brevis and flexor digitorum brevis are located deep in the foot and flex the toes.

Plantar Fascia

The plantar fascia is a strong fibrous tissue, thick in the center and thin on the sides. It originates deep within the plantar surface of the calcaneum and represents the distal part of the plantaris (**Fig. 3**) which has become separated from the rest of the muscle during evolution because of the heel enlargement. It functions in providing attachment to the skin of the sole, protecting the deeper structures and helping the longitudinal arch of the foot.

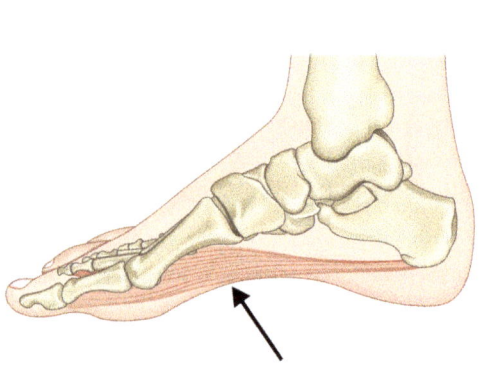
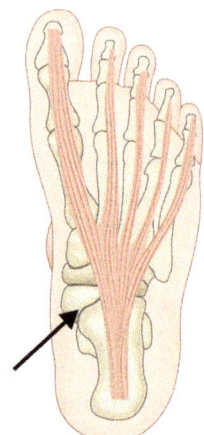

FIG. 3: Plantar fascia.

The superficial fascia has fibrous and dense bands, which bind the skin to the plantar aponeurosis. It divides the subcutaneous fat into small tight compartments which serve as water cushions reinforcing the spring effect of the arches of the foot during walking, running, and jumping.

During walking, when the foot rolls off the ground, the toes dorsiflex and pull on this fascia. This motion tightens the plantar fascia and thereby supports the arch of the foot by maintaining the distance between the calcaneum and the metatarsal heads. This phenomenon is known as *windlass mechanism*. This stiff and relatively impermeable covering helps to protect the muscles of the foot.

The skin of the sole is thick for protection and firmly adherent to the underlying plantar aponeurosis and crease. These features increase the efficiency of the grip of the sole on the ground.[3]

Arches of the Foot

The foot acts as a pliable platform to support the body weight in the upright posture and as a lever to propel the body forward in walking, running, or jumping. To meet these requirements, the foot is designed in the form of elastic arches or springs. These arches are segmented so they can best sustain the stresses of weight and thrusts. The general shape of the articulated tarsal and metatarsal bones of the foot is that of a half dome, concave inferiorly. When the feet are together, the two half domes form a single dome. The rim of each half dome consists of the heel, lateral border of the foot, and the heads of the metatarsal heads. The footprint of a bare foot is formed by the skin covering these parts of the foot when it comes in contact with the ground. The arches are present right from birth; however, they are masked in infants by the excessive amount of fat in the soles.[4]

The arches may be classified as:
- Longitudinal:
  - Medial
  - Lateral
- Transverse:
  - Anterior
  - Posterior

The arches consist of anterior and posterior ends where it is attached to the bones, pillars formed by the metatarsals. Intersegmental ties are the ligaments that hold the different segments of the arch together and tie-beams connect two ends of an arch.

The medial longitudinal arch is considerably higher, more mobile and resilient than the lateral arch. On the lateral side, it is nearly flat (**Fig. 4**).

The anterior transverse arch is formed by the heads of the five metatarsal bones. It is a complete arch as the heads of both the first and the fifth metatarsals come in contact with the ground and form the two ends of the arch. The posterior arch is incomplete as only the lateral end comes in contact with the ground forming half a dome which is completed by a similar half dome in the opposite foot.

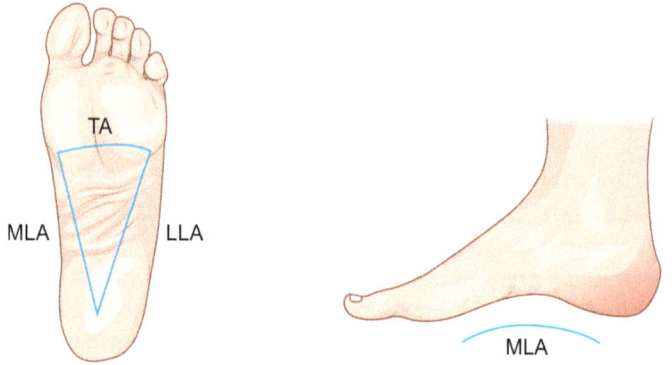

(LLA: lateral longitudinal arch; MLA: medial longitudinal arch; TA: transverse arch)

FIG. 4: Arches of the foot.

The absence or collapse of the arches leads to *pes planus* (flat foot) which can give rise to the following conditions:
- Loss of spring in the foot leading to a clumsy, shuffling gait
- Loss of shock-absorbing function making the foot more liable to trauma and osteoarthritis
- Loss of concavity of the sole leads to compression of the nerves and blood vessels causing metatarsalgia and vascular disturbances[5]

Nerve Supply

There are five nerves that pass beyond the ankle joint to supply the foot (**Fig. 5**). These nerves are branches of the sciatic and the femoral nerves, originating from the lumbosacral plexus.
1. *Saphenous nerve*: Originates from the femoral nerve. It runs over the medial aspect of the ankle and supplies sensation to the inside of the foot.
2. *Sural nerve*: This is a sensory branch of the tibial nerve. It runs below the knee to the lateral aspect of the foot. It is very superficial at the level of the posterolateral ankle and continues distally to provide sensation to the outside of the foot.
3. *Superficial peroneal nerve*: This is a branch of the common peroneal nerve and innervates the lateral compartment muscles. Though this nerve is both motor and sensory, below the ankle, it only supplies sensations to the lateral aspect of the foot.
4. *Deep peroneal nerve*: This is the other branch of common peroneal nerve which supplies the anterior compartment of the leg. It does not have any motor supply beyond the ankle. Its terminal branch provides sensations to the first web space.
5. *Posterior tibial nerve*: This is a branch of the tibial nerve that runs in the back of the calf supplying the muscles of the deep and superficial posterior compartments. This nerve runs behind the medial malleolus and divides into the medial and lateral plantar nerves. These supply sensation to the entire sole of the foot.[6]

Anatomy and Biomechanics of the Diabetic Foot

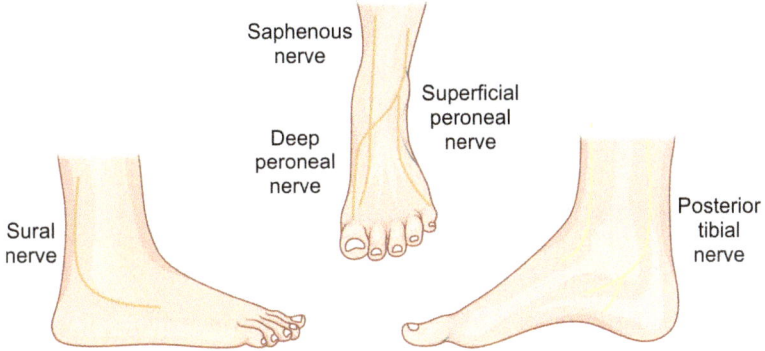

FIG. 5: Nerve supply of foot and ankle.

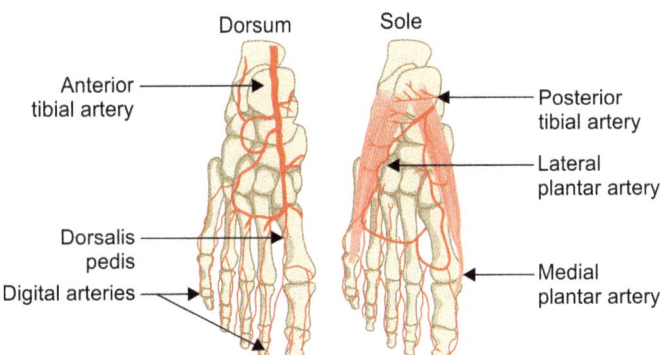

FIG. 6: Blood supply of the foot.

Blood Supply

The three primary sources of blood supply to the foot and ankle are the posterior tibial, the dorsalis pedis (anterior tibial), and the peroneal arteries (**Fig. 6**).

The *posterior tibial artery* is the larger of the two branches of popliteal artery and is the main blood supply to the superficial and deep compartments of the leg. In the ankle, it passes behind the medial malleolus and in the foot, it divides into lateral and medial plantar arteries. These two terminal branches are the chief arteries of sole of the foot.

The anterior *tibial artery* is the smaller of the two branches of popliteal artery and supplies the muscles of the anterior compartment of the leg. In the foot, it continues as dorsalis pedis artery and terminates into deep plantar arch.

The *peroneal artery* is the largest branch of posterior tibial artery and supplies the posterior and lateral compartments of the leg. It divides at the ankle to give rise to posterolateral malleolar artery and a communicating branch. Its terminal branch in the foot is lateral calcaneal artery.

Blood supply to the plantar aspect of the foot and the toes comes from the plantar arch that is formed by the anastomosis of lateral plantar artery and the dorsalis pedis artery. It gives off plantar metatarsal arteries and plantar digital arteries.

The dorsal venous arch drains into the great saphenous and short saphenous veins.[7]

BIOMECHANICS

Motions of the Ankle and Foot Complex

The foot has the characteristics of a triple axial joint which allows it to assume any position during walking, particularly during rotational movements on an uneven surface. The three main axes of movement converge in the area of the talus (**Fig. 7**). Though all the joints are involved to some extent in walking, the ankle joint, although a hinge joint, forms the main joint of locomotion.

The movements permitted at the joints of the ankle and foot are:
- *Plantar flexion and dorsiflexion*: Occur in a sagittal lane around a coronal axis (**Fig. 8**). This movement is at the ankle joint.
- *Inversion and eversion*: This movement occurs mainly at subtalar joint, in the frontal plane around a longitudinal axis (**Fig. 9**). The intertarsal, TMT, and inter-metatarsal joints permit gliding and rotatory movements which jointly bring about inversion and eversion.
- *Adduction and abduction*: This occurs in the transverse plane around a vertical axis. The metatarsophalangeal joints are similar to metacarpal joints of the hand. They permit flexion, extension, adduction, and abduction of the toes.
- *Pronation and supination*: These motions occur around an axis that lies at an angle to each of the axes for "cardinal" motions of dorsiflexion/plantar flexion,

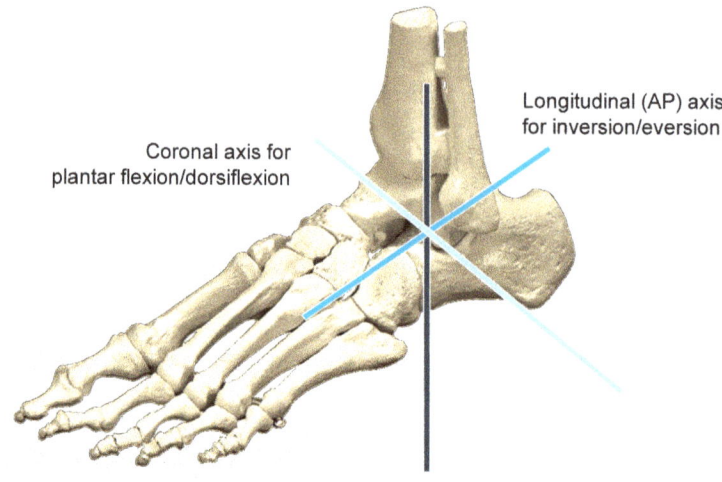

FIG. 7: Joint axis.

Anatomy and Biomechanics of the Diabetic Foot

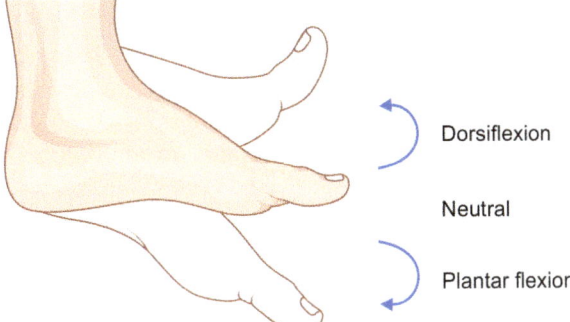

FIG. 8: Ankle joint range of motion.

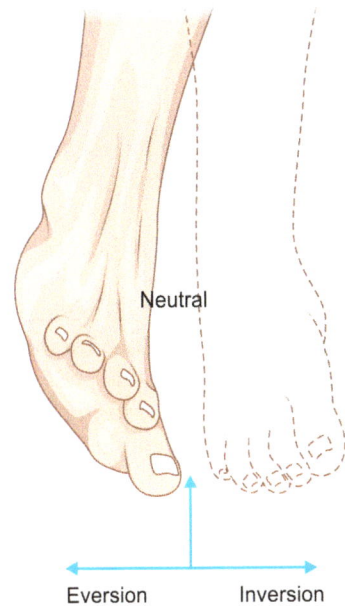

FIG. 9: Movement at the subtalar joint.

inversion/eversion, and abduction/adduction. Pronation and supination are terms used to describe "composite" motions that have components of, or are coupled to, each of the cardinal motions. Pronation is a motion about an axis that results in coupled motions of dorsiflexion, eversion, and abduction. Supination is a motion about an axis that results in coupled motions of plantarflexion, inversion, and adduction. The proportional contribution that each of the coupled motions makes to pronation/supination is dependent on and varies with the angle of the pronation/supination joint axis.
- The interphalangeal joints permit flexion and extension of the distal phalanges.[8]

Foot Dynamics and Gait

Strength and resilience are the main features of the foot. Strength is obtained by the tarsal and the big toe bones bound together by powerful ligaments. By binding the first metatarsal to those of the other toes, mobility is restricted when compared with the hand. Resilience is obtained by the presence of multiple joints, each of which have limited movement, except for those concerned with inversion and eversion of the foot. The arrangement of the bones in an arch, held together by plantar ligaments and a strong tie-beam (plantar aponeurosis), also contribute toward resilience. The plantar aponeurosis binds the ends of the arch together, and has altered tension in different positions of the foot. While standing, weight is supported on the heel and on the metatarsal heads (mainly the first metatarsal), and to a lesser extent on the lateral border of the sole of the foot. Similarly, while thrusting the foot, the force is carried principally on the head of the first metatarsal and the big toe. The remaining metatarsals and toes are relatively weaker, and act as stabilizing structures. Without these, the foot is rendered unstable, giving only a two-point contact with the ground: on the calcaneus and the ball of the big toe. The arch shape of the foot has the added advantage of giving protection to the structures in the sole, which would otherwise be subjected to pressure. The presence of the sesamoid bones on the head of the first metatarsal (on plantar surface), resist pressure on it. Sesamoid bones also transmit the pull of the small muscles of the big toe (without subjecting them to pressure) through a tunnel between them, which allows the long flexor tendon to pass through to reach the distal phalanx.

The gait cycle consists of the stance and the swing phases. The stance phase is further divided into subphases (**Fig. 10**). Initial contact (also known as *heel strike*) occurs at the onset of the gait cycle. During this phase, the foot touches the ground and the calcaneum bears all the weight. Due to the strike, there is increased thrust, which lasts for a short duration. After initial contact, foot flat (loading response phase) is the first instance at which the foot is flat on the ground. During this, the pressure falls

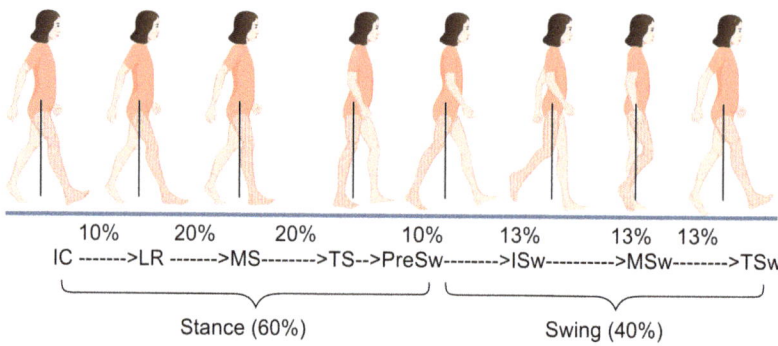

(IC: initial contact; LR: loading response; MS: mid-stance; TS: terminal stance; PreSw: preswing; ISw: initial swing; MSw: mid-swing; TSw: terminal swing)

FIG. 10: Phases of gait cycle.

on the talus, dividing along the anterior of the foot and pillars of the arch. The lateral border of the foot also takes the strain, transmitting the weight through the cuboid and the base of the fifth metatarsal. At midstance, the foot comes in total contact with the ground. The body's weight is borne by the calcaneum, the base of the metatarsal, and the heads of all the metatarsals.

Push-off phase begins with heel-off and is followed by toe-off. At the onset of push-off, the heel begins to leave the ground (heel-off). The gastrocnemius muscle pulls the calcaneum upwards, acting as a fulcrum. This exerts a pull on the bowstring of the sole muscles and ligaments, thereby supporting the pillars of the arch. Only the metatarsal heads rest on the ground. Contraction of the long flexors of the toes gives the final thrust which pushes the body forward, taking weight off the foot, initiating the swing phase.[9]

While walking, the foot is therefore required to be initially unstable to adapt to the terrain and also to absorb shock. Whereas, during the propulsion phase, the foot has to be stable in order to function as a lever. Foot flexibility and rigidity are mainly controlled with pronation and supination of the subtalar and midtarsal joints. Subtalar joint pronation following heel strike is a major shock-absorbing mechanism. Limited joint mobility (LJM) or structural abnormality can compromise flexibility and shock absorption, thereby placing increased stress on the plantar surface of the skin. In addition, limited ankle dorsiflexion could result in increased pressure on the forefoot, particularly during the late stance phase, which is caused by an early heel rise or compensatory pronation.

Foot Changes in Diabetes and Peripheral Neuropathy

Diabetic peripheral neuropathy leads not only to a reduction in, or loss of protective sensation (sensory neuropathy) but also to changes in architecture of the foot (motor neuropathy), as well as dryness of the skin (autonomic neuropathy). This leads to callus formation and changes in plantar pressures. Along with neuropathy, there are other pathophysiological mechanisms such as peripheral vascular disease, foot deformity, higher foot pressures, and poor glycemic control which contribute to ulceration. Diabetic neuropathy and peripheral vascular disease, however, are the main etiological factors in predisposition of foot ulceration and poor healing. These two factors may act alone, together, or in combination with other factors. Trauma plays an important role in causing tissue breakdown, in addition to neuropathy and vascular disease.[10]

Biomechanical Aspects of Foot Ulceration

Common sites where ulcers form are under the plantar surface of the toes, forefoot, and midfoot, followed by the dorsal surface of the toes and heel. Changes in foot architecture, affecting foot function and causing deformities are usually responsible for excessive pressures. They commonly occur at sites with bony prominences, such as at the first metatarsal head.

If similar pressures occurred in a person with intact or adequate sensation, there will be perception of pain, thereby avoiding the pressure. However, in a person with loss of protective sensation, there is no warning of excessive pressure or tissue damage and persistent localized pressures lead to skin breakdown or ulceration. Therefore, excessive and/or repetitive pressure can be one of the major factors for breakdown of skin.

Three mechanisms can be seen for the occurrence of these pressures:
1. Duration of pressures
2. Magnitude of pressures
3. Repetition of pressure

The first mechanism includes relatively low pressures applied for a long period of time causing ischemia. Prolonged ischemia leads to cell death and wound formation. An inverse relationship exists between time and pressure. High pressures take a relatively short time to cause ulceration, whereas low pressures take a relatively long time. Thus, ulceration can develop at very low pressures, but may take a few days to occur. This type of offending pressure and resulting ulcers can occur with ill-fitting footwear, improperly fitted orthotics, or prolonged resting of a heel on a bed or footrest.

The second mechanism of tissue injury includes high pressures acting for a short-time period. This injury only happens if a large force is applied to a relatively small area of skin. This happens, for example, if a person steps on a nail, pebble, or piece of glass, which is not uncommon for diabetic patients with neuropathy.

The third mechanism of injury comes from repetitions of pressure, which in turn leads to mechanical fatigue. This is defined as failure of a structure or biological tissue to maintain integrity at submaximal level when subjected to repeated bouts of loading. This type of injury occurs in the insensitive skin and subcutaneous tissue of the neuropathic foot. The body will respond to repeated high pressures or microtrauma with callus formation in order to protect the skin from further damage. However, if callus formation becomes excessive, it will contribute to higher pressures and therefore must be removed at a regular interval. Thus, not only is the magnitude of the plantar pressure important in causing foot ulceration but also several other factors such as the rate of increase of pressure, duration of high pressure, and the frequency of applied pressure to the skin should be taken into account. In addition, although foot pressures may be high during a barefoot pressure assessment, it is important to keep in mind that it is the combination of footwear, lifestyle factors, tissue characteristics, foot pressures, and level of physical activity, which contribute to the development of foot ulceration.

Limited Joint Mobility

Joint mobility is defined as the range of motion of a joint and is related to age and gender. LJM of the foot and ankle can cause an increase in plantar pressure in diabetic and thereby related to foot ulceration. Collagen abnormalities and non-enzymatic glycation of soft tissue that occur in diabetes, resulting in thickening of skin, tendons, ligaments and joint capsules, reducing tissue flexibility, contribute to this problem.

Joint mobility of the subtalar joint is affected in the ulcerated foot compared with the non-ulcerated foot in diabetic neuropathic patients. Also, ankle dorsiflexion and subtalar range of motion are reduced in diabetic patients with a history of plantar ulceration compared to patients without ulceration and nondiabetics. In addition, ulceration of the great toe has been associated with a reduced range of motion at the first metatarsal pharyngeal joint (MTPJ). Foot ulceration caused due to other etiological factors can also be a reason for stiffening of the joints as opposed to LJM causing foot ulceration. One of the interventions used for managing foot ulcers is total contact casting for off-loading the foot. This, along with advise to patients to minimize their level of physical activity ulcer healing are two factors which are quite likely to compromise joint mobility as well.[2]

Plantar Tissue Thickness and Foot Ulceration

Plantar tissue thickness is strongly associated with plantar pressure, indicating a close relation between the amount of cushioning (soft tissue) available and the pressure distribution at the forefoot. Changes of the plantar fat pad have also been seen in the form of a non-specific fibrotic process beneath the metatarsal head in patients with diabetic neuropathy. This fibrotic tissue affects the intrinsic biomechanical properties of the plantar fat pad to act as a shock absorber and dissipate increased plantar pressures associated with neuropathy. Prominent metatarsal heads have been attributed to weakness of the intrinsic muscles of the foot, leading to toe deformities in patients with diabetic neuropathy. Fat cushions under metatarsal heads, which are imbedded in the flexor tendons, migrate distally with clawing and hammering of the toes, leaving the metatarsal heads relatively unprotected. Atrophy of these muscles has been seen as fatty infiltration in plantar muscles of diabetic patients with a history of foot ulceration. However, foot muscle atrophy in patients with diabetic neuropathy results in different areas experiencing different pressures and therefore the threshold for pressure changes.

Foot Type and Ulceration

Feet with abnormal alignment of the forefoot or rearfoot exhibit a different loading pattern than normally aligned feet. Both non-diabetic and diabetic persons with pes planus (everted rearfoot, inverted forefoot and low arch) have shown to have greater peak pressures than non-diabetic normal feet (a neutral rearfoot and forefoot with normal arch morphology). Persons with an uncompensated forefoot varus or forefoot valgus (inverted or everted forefoot) develop ulcers located at the first or fifth MTH. Similarly, calcaneovarus (inverted heel position) has been associated with lateral ulcers, whereas calcaneovalgus (everted heel position) is associated with medial ulcers (**Figs. 11A** and **B**). Thus, high pressures may not just be caused by the effects of diabetes; but diabetics with preexisting foot-type characteristics that differ from the normal are more likely to develop high foot pressures and ulceration than diabetic patients with normal foot morphology.

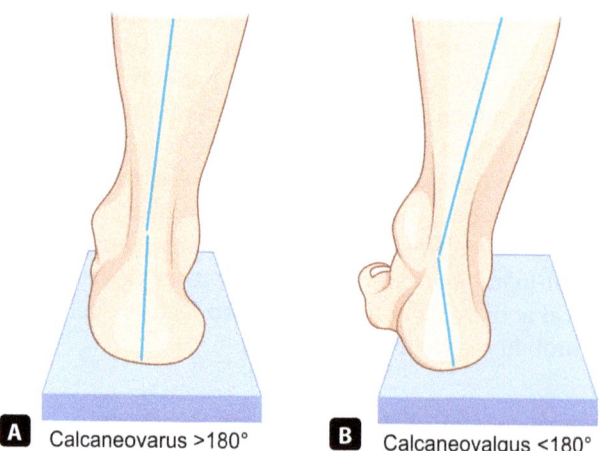

A Calcaneovarus >180°   B Calcaneovalgus <180°

FIGS. 11A AND B: (A) Calcaneovarus; and (B) Calcaneovalgus.

An understanding of the biomechanics and basic anatomy of the foot is essential for clinicians managing patients with diabetes. This helps in planning appropriate intervention and prevention of major morbidities and mortality. Early implementation of biomechanical intervention will in turn reduce the rate of amputations and better quality of life for the individual.

REFERENCES

1. Chan CW, Rudins A. Foot biomechanics during walking and running. Mayo Clin Proc. 1994;69(5):448-61.
2. van Schie CHM. A review of the biomechanics of the diabetic foot. Int J Low Extrem Wounds. 2005;4(3):160-70.
3. Xiong S, Goonetilleke RS, Witana CP, Weerasinghe TW, Au EYL. Foot arch characterization: a review, a new metric, and a comparison. J Am Podiatr Med Assoc. 2010;100(1):14-24.
4. Donatelli RA. Normal biomechanics of the foot and ankle. J Orthop Sports Phys Ther. 1985;7(3):91-5.
5. Kenhub. (2021). Arches of the foot: Anatomy. [online] Available from: https://www.kenhub.com/en/library/anatomy/arches-of-the-foot. [Last accessed November 2021].
6. Tang A, Bordoni B. Anatomy, bony pelvis and lower limb, foot nerves. In: StatPearls. Treasure Island (FL): StatPearls Publishing; 2021.
7. Robinson S-A, Carlin R. Anatomy, bony pelvis and lower limb, foot dorsalis pedis artery. In: StatPearls Treasure Island (FL): StatPearls Publishing; 2021.
8. Kim PJ. Biomechanics of the Diabetic Foot: Consideration in Limb Salvage. Adv Wound Care. 2013;2(3):107-11.
9. Pol F, Baharlouei H, Taheri A, Menz HB, Forghany S. Foot and ankle biomechanics during walking in older adults: A systematic review and meta-analysis of observational studies. Gait Posture. 2021;89:14-24.
10. Kuo AD, Donelan JM. Dynamic principles of gait and their clinical implications. Physical Therapy. 2010;90(2):157-74.

CHAPTER 3

PAUL BRAND

Dr Paul Brand was born in 1914 and grew up in the Kolli Hills of Tamil Nadu in India. He is a world-renowned leprosy surgeon and specialist in orthopedics. He completed his medical training from London University. Dr Brand returned to India in 1946, to teach surgery at the Christian Medical College and Hospital, Vellore. During the time, leprosy (Hansen's Disease) was stigmatized and very little was known about the disease. Dr Brand was determined to help people with leprosy and hence researched the topic in great detail. He discovered that the 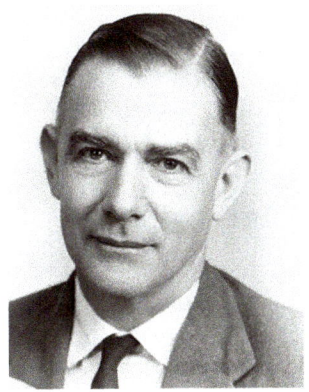 damage was not caused directly by bacteria; which was the common belief of physicians at the time. Instead, it was caused by ordinary, often small, injuries which happened because the person with Hansen's disease could not feel pain. This was a novel finding which eventually changed the lives of many. Drawing on his experience of treating patients with polio and paralyzed hands due to war-injuries, from the Second World War, he pioneered tendon transfer techniques with leprosy patients, and opened up new possibilities of disability prevention and rehabilitation.

Peripheral Neuropathy: Clinical Approach

*Jinson Paul, Shivendra Verma, Kripa Elizabeth Cherian, Flory Christina I,
B Vinod Jacob, Felix Jebasingh K, Nihal Thomas*

CASE 1

A 58-year-old gentleman who was known to have type 2 diabetes mellitus (T2DM) since the age of 48 years, presented with burning sensation and paresthesias of both lower limbs up to the level of the mid-calf for the last 6 months. He was on regular oral antidiabetic medications. His blood glucose levels were persistently high for many years despite taking regular medications. His glycated hemoglobin (HbA1c) level done 3 months prior to this visit to the hospital was 12%. He was on pregabalin at a dose of 150 mg over the last 3 months without much symptomatic relief in pain in his lower limb. He was advised to use premixed insulin for his glycemic control in the past, but was hesitant to use it.

On examination, he had severe bilateral sensory polyneuropathy, normal motor system, normal deep tendon reflexes, normal autonomic function tests (AFTs), and normal cranial nerves examination. He had bilateral moderate nonproliferative diabetic retinopathy (NPDR) without Clinically Significant Macular Edema (CSME). His repeat biochemistry tests showed HbA1c of 12%, elevated urinary microalbumin, and normal liver and renal function tests.

What would be the further work up and treatment which may be offered for this patient?

CASE 2

A 40-year-old gentleman with a history of diabetes mellitus (DM) for the last 2 years on oral antidiabetic medications presented with recent onset paresthesias of both feet and hands. On examination, his deep tendon reflexes were absent. He did not have evidence of diabetic retinopathy or diabetic nephropathy. His HbA1c was 6.5%, and renal, liver, and thyroid function tests were normal.

INTRODUCTION

The peripheral neuropathy associated with DM is the most common microvascular complication due to persistent hyperglycemic state. Diabetic neuropathy (DN) causes significant morbidity and mortality predominantly due to pain and decreased sensation on the peripheries. The peripheral nervous system can be classified as shown in **Figure 1**. The prevalence of DN varies across the world owing to the variable of DM as well as the variable criteria used in diagnosing DN.

In an outpatient study conducted across four institutions in India including our center, a prevalence of DN was between 14 and 17% using a nylon monofilament was demonstrated. Moreover, it also noted that the prediabetic status is a predictor for an early occurrence of DN.

Diabetic neuropathy induced complications are a major reason for hospitalizations and are also responsible for more than half of the nontraumatic amputations among hospitalized patients. In addition, neurological complications are seen in type 1 diabetes mellitus (T1DM) and in other congenital and acquired forms of DM.

There are different types of sensory nerve fibers (**Table 1**). The major complication associated with peripheral sensory neuropathy is foot ulceration. Many of the ulcers are a precursor for gangrene and subsequent minor or major amputations. The studies have noted that the underlying peripheral neuropathy increases the risk of any kind of amputations by 1.7-fold. The risk increased by 12-fold if there is a deformity (due

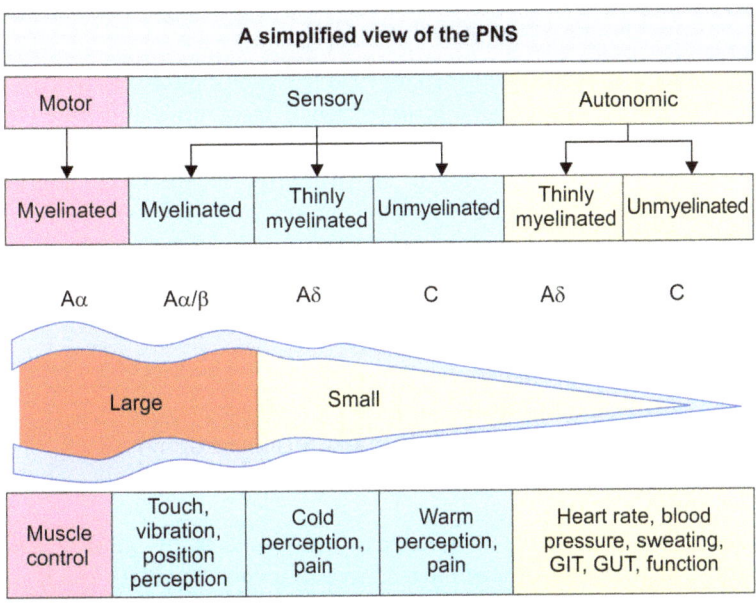

(GIT: gastrointestinal tract; GUT: genitourinary tract; PNS: peripheral nervous system)

FIG. 1: Classification of peripheral nerves based on myelination.

TABLE 1: Different types of sensory nerve fibers.

Sensory neuron fiber types				
General classification	Nerve classification	Fiber diameter velocity	Myelination	Sensory modalities
Aα	I	13–20 μm 120–160 m/s	Yes	Proprioception
Aβ	II	6–12 μm 75–35 m/s	Yes	• Proprioception • Superficial touch • Deep touch • Vibration
Aδ	III	1–5 μm 30–06 m/s	Yes	• Pain • Temperature (cool)
C	IV	0.2–1.5 μm 2–0.5 m/s	No	• Pain • Temperature (warm) • Itch

to motor neuropathy), and increased manifold to 36 times if there is a history of ulcer in the past.[1]

CLASSIFICATION

There are various classifications available for DN.

The main groups of neurologic disturbances in DM include the following:
- Subclinical neuropathy, which is determined by abnormalities in electrodiagnostic and quantitative sensory testing
- Diffuse clinical neuropathy with distal symmetric sensori-motor and autonomic syndromes
    - Sensory or sensorimotor polyneuropathy
    - Selective small-fiber polyneuropathy
    - Autonomic neuropathy
- *Focal syndromes*:
    - Truncal mononeuropathy
    - Mononeuritis multiplex
    - Asymmetric lower limb motor neuropathy (amyotrophy)
    - Cranial neuropathy
- Mixed forms

Subclinical neuropathy is diagnosed when there is no clinical evidence of neuropathy, however has abnormal electrodiagnostic tests with decreased nerve conduction velocity (NCV) or decreased amplitude; quantitative sensory tests (QSTs) showing altered vibration perception, tactile or touch and temperature perception and AFTs revealing sympathetic and parasympathetic nerve dysfunction.[2,3]

RISK FACTORS FOR PERIPHERAL NEUROPATHY

The following are the risk factors for development of diabetes-related peripheral neuropathy:[4]

Those with major impact are:
- Poor glycemic control
- Long-standing DM
- Damage to blood vessels
- Alcohol consumption

Those with minor impact are:
- Autoimmune factors
- Genetic susceptibility
- Smoking
- Low high-density lipoprotein (HDL)
- Cardiovascular disease

The duration of DM was found to be a major risk factor for neuropathy with the odds of developing neuropathy in patients who had DM for more than 15 years' duration being 8.03 [95% confidence interval (CI) 5.96–10.8, $p < 0.001$] when compared with a duration less than 5 years. In this study, it was found that the increasing age, presence of dyslipidemia, and the presence of other microvascular complications were found to be significantly associated with peripheral neuropathy.[4]

PATHOGENESIS OF PERIPHERAL NEUROPATHY (FIG. 2)

Metabolic Hypothesis

Chronic hyperglycemia induces peripheral nerve injury through multiple pathways, one of which is due to increased influx of polyol which is regulated by aldose reductase, commonly known as polyol pathway. Another hypothesis is that injury to the endoneurium of peripheral nerves is caused by the increased deposition of advanced glycation end-products (AGEs).[5] Yet another mechanism of hyperglycemia contributing to peripheral neuropathy is by oxidative stress-induced free radicals generated in the glycolytic process.[6]

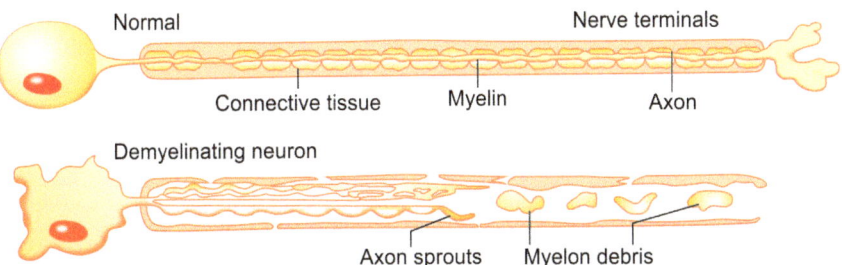

FIG. 2: Peripheral nerve damage in diabetes mellitus (DM) (normal nerve fibers vs. damaged nerve fibers in DM).

Immune Hypothesis

Antiphospholipid antibodies and autoantibodies to gangliosides were also detected in patients with DN making this a potential pathology in developing DN.

Microvascular Hypothesis

Microvascular insufficiency due to vascular insufficiency of vasovasorum, contributed by increase in wall thickness, hyalinization of basal lamina of vessels, and impaired vasoconstriction and vasodilatation, leads to nerve ischemia.

Neurotrophic Hypothesis

Deficiency of neurotrophic factors such as nerve growth factor (NGF), neurotrophin-3/4/5, and insulin-like growth factor (IGF)-1 is noted in patients with DN.[7]

CLINICAL EVALUATION

History

The neuropathic symptoms are divided into focal and diffuse forms. The latter is far more common than the other.

Diffuse Neuropathies

One should look for specific motor and sensory symptoms in patients as it helps in understanding the underlying nerves at fault. This can be understood from the following (**Flowchart 1**).

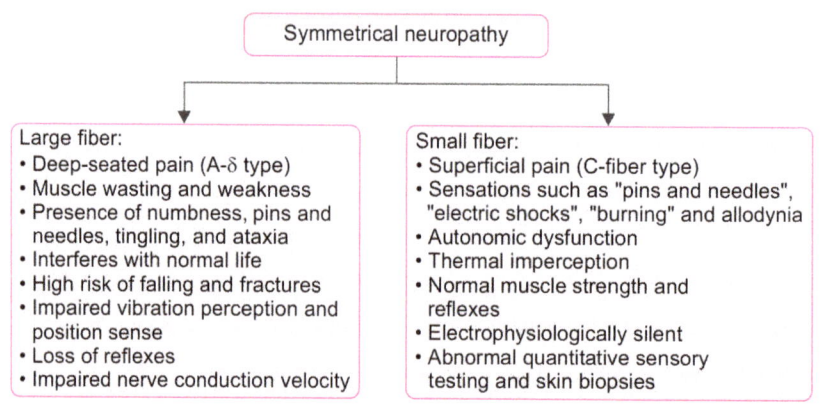

FLOWCHART 1: Differences in clinical presentations of large- and small-fiber neuropathies.

Acute Painful Neuropathy

Some patients with DM present with acute symptoms, which persist for <6 months and are associated with moderate-to-severe pain. Pain due to sensory neuropathy is exacerbated during night time, often felt more in the feet than in the hands. Due to nocturnal pain, most often the patient complaints of sleep disturbance and insomnia. The pain can be of burning, stabbing, paresthesias, pins and needles prick sensation, and tingling in nature.

The possibilities to be considered in such scenario are as follows:
- Insulin neuritis
- Rapid correction of blood glucose
- Chronic alcohol consumption
- Associated amyloidosis and multiple myeloma
- Human immunodeficiency virus (HIV) infection
- Heavy metal poisoning (e.g., arsenic)
- Fabrys disease

Chronic Painful Neuropathy

Chronic painful neuropathy is another entity, late in onset, occurs after years of diagnosis of DM; wherein the debilitating pain persists >6 months.

Many of them in the long term can have absence of pain which is not due to improvement of symptoms, but due to neuronal loss.

Hyperalgesia is increased pain perception even for normal stimuli. Allodynia is pain perceived by a stimulus that is not usually painful.

C and Aδ fibers are responsible for burning and pricking sensations. Also, Aβ fibers are responsible for dysesthesias, paresthesias, or allodynia. The differential diagnosis for painful DN is given in **Table 2**.

Large-fiber Neuropathies

Large-fiber neuropathies involve sensory or motor nerves. These neuropathies have more signs than symptoms. Vibration perception, position sense, and cold thermal perception are altered in fiber neuropathies. These myelinated, rapidly conducting fibers tend to affect toes more than the fingers as it is length dependent fibers which are more evident in electromyography (EMG). Alteration in these fibers causes cotton feel in the feet while walking and in severe cases, nondiscrimination of shapes and difficulty in turning the papers in the books. The differences between large- and small-fiber neuropathies are given in **Flowchart 1**.

Clinical presentation of large-fiber neuropathies includes the following:
- Impaired vibration perception (often the first objective evidence) and position sense
- Depressed tendon reflexes
- A delta-type deep-seated gnawing, dull, like a toothache in the bones of the feet, or even crushing or cramp-like pain

TABLE 2: Differentials for painful diabetic peripheral neuropathy.

Condition	Key characteristics and differentiating features
Osteoarthritis	Can be secondary to DM, but pain is usually gradual in onset and in one or two joints. Pain worsens with exercise and improves with rest
Plantar fasciitis	Pain in the plantar region of the foot. Tenderness along the plantar fascia when the ankle is dorsiflexed. Shooting or burning in the heel with each step. Worsening pain with prolonged activity is often associated with a calcaneal spur on radiography
Tarsal tunnel syndrome	Caused by entrapment of the posterior tibial nerve. Pain and numbness radiate from beneath the medial malleolus to the sole of the foot. Clinical examination includes percussion, palpation for possible soft tissue matter, nerve conduction studies, and MRI
Claudication pain	Doppler ultrasonography confirms clinical diagnosis of arterial occlusion. Patients with diabetes may present with normal extremities and absent foot pulses. Peripheral arterial occlusion with underlying atherosclerosis. Usually intermittent, worsened by walking; remits with rest; other signs or symptoms suggest arterial insufficiency
Charcot neuroarthropathy	May result from osteopenia caused by increased blood flow following repeated minor trauma in individuals with diabetic neuropathy. A warm to hot foot with an increased blood flow, decreased warm sensory perception, and vibration detection
Radiculopathy	Can be caused by diabetes, but can also result from arthritis or metastatic disease. Neurologic examination and imaging can localize lesion site. Pain can occur in the thorax, extremities, shoulder, or arm, depending on the site of the lesion
Morton's neuroma	Benign neuroma formation on the third plantar interdigital nerve. Generally unilateral, more frequent in women. Pain elicited when pressure is applied with the thumb between the first and fourth metatarsal heads

(MRI: magnetic resonance imaging)

- Sensory ataxia (waddling gait)
- Wasting of small muscles of feet with hammer toes (intrinsic muscles in the feet)
- Shortening of the Achilles tendon with pes equinus
- Increased blood flow (warm foot)

Proximal Motor Neuropathies

The synonyms for proximal neuropathy are femoral neuropathy, diabetic amyotrophy,[6] and diabetic neuropathic cachexia.

Proximal motor neuropathy has discrete symptoms and signs:
- Primarily affects the elderly, commonly after fifth decade of life
- Gradual or abrupt onset

- Starts with one leg and progress to other leg
- Initial symptom is pain in the thighs, hips, or buttocks
- Subsequent sign is proximal myopathy.
- Heel or toe standing is usually normal though having proximal muscles weakness.
- Spontaneous or provoked fasciculations
- EMG reveals features of lumbosacral plexopathy

Though this is commonly associated with DM, other causes such as chronic inflammatory demyelinating polyneuropathy (CIDP), monoclonal gammopathy of unknown significance (MGUS), circulating GM1 antibodies, and antibodies to neuronal cells and inflammatory vasculitis should be kept in mind.

If demyelination predominates in EMG, the causes other than DM has to be investigated further as the treatment option differs from DM-related femoral neuropathy.

Asymmetric Neuropathies
Focal Neuropathies
- *Mononeuropathy*:
  - Usually in older population
  - Generally acute with pain
  - It can involve truncal and cranial nerves (III and VI)
  - Self-limiting and resolving in 6–8 weeks
  - Usually due to vessel occlusion
  - *Treatment*: Symptomatic for pain and physiotherapy
- *Entrapment neuropathy*:
  - Starts slowly and progresses slowly.
  - Commonly involves median (carpel tunnel), ulnar, radial, femoral, and lateral cutaneous nerve of thigh.
  - Treated with splints, nonsteroidal anti-inflammatory drugs (NSAIDs), and local injection
  - In some cases, surgery to decompress

Mononeuropathies must be distinguished from entrapment syndromes, which start slowly, progress, and persist without intervention.

Cranial Neuropathy
In patients with DM, the most commonly involved cranial nerve is oculomotor nerve (3rd cranial nerve) followed by trochlear (4th nerve) and facial (7th) nerves. Oculomotor (3rd cranial nerve) with pupillary sparing is the hallmark of diabetes-related cranial mononeuropathy. Ischemia of the nerves due to occlusion of vasovasorum is the pathophysiology behind the occurrence of mononeuropathy. The pupillary fibers are peripherally located and hence these fibers are spared; thereby the pupils are not affected in patients with DM and oculomotor palsy.

EVALUATION OF THE PATIENT

Monofilament Testing

Von Frey in 19th century made the first monofilament from horse hairs to test the pressure sensation. Later Semmes and Weinstein used similar technique in studying the peripheral neuropathy in brain damaged patients. The monofilament was subsequently used in Hansen disease in the middle of 20th century. The monofilaments which are used at present are made from nylon fibers.

How to use 10 g Monofilament

The 10 g monofilament is a simple tool to measure the loss of protective sensation (LOPS). The color coding for different monofilament is given in **Box 1** and **Figure 3**. In our institution, we also use 2 g and 4 g as it can detect early peripheral neuropathy.

It is also important to give rest to the monofilament for 24 hours after having been used in 10–15 patients on a single day and it has to be replaced after being used in 70–90 patients. Monofilaments should be replaced immediately if they are damaged or bent.

BOX 1: Color coding for monofilaments.	
• 0.5 g = Light blue	• 4.0 g = Red
• 2.0 g = Purple	• 10.0 g = Orange

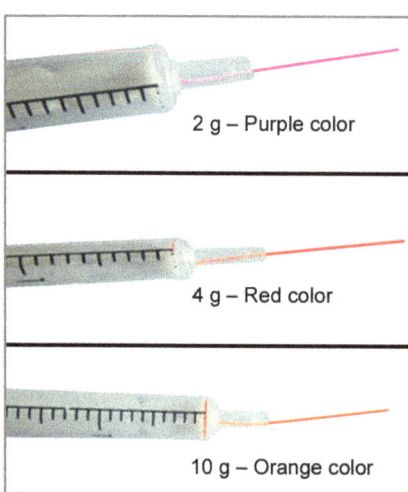

FIG. 3: Different types of monofilament.

Peripheral Neuropathy: Clinical Approach

Method of Using the Monofilament

The patients should be explained about the procedure by applying the monofilament in the upper limb and make the patient aware of the sensation. This helps in warming up the patient.

- Gently apply a force in such a way that the filament takes a "c" shape or buckles (**Figs. 4A** and **B**).
- The total time taken for the approach to skin contact, and withdrawal of the filament should be around 2 seconds.
- Avoid applying the monofilament over callous, scar, ulcer, necrotic tissue, gangrene, and its perimeter area. One should take care that they do not slide or flick the skin with the monofilament while applying.
- We use 10 sites in our institution for the detection of peripheral neuropathy (**Fig. 5**)

  Loss of protective sensation (LOPS) = No sensation in more than 6 sites

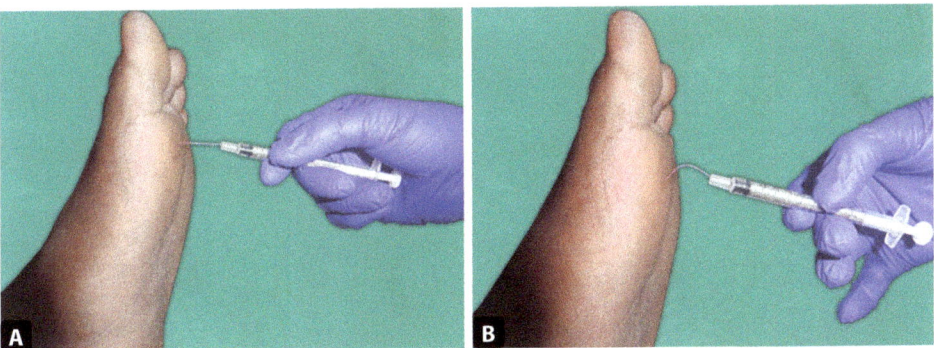

FIGS. 4A AND B: The appropriate method of using monofilaments.

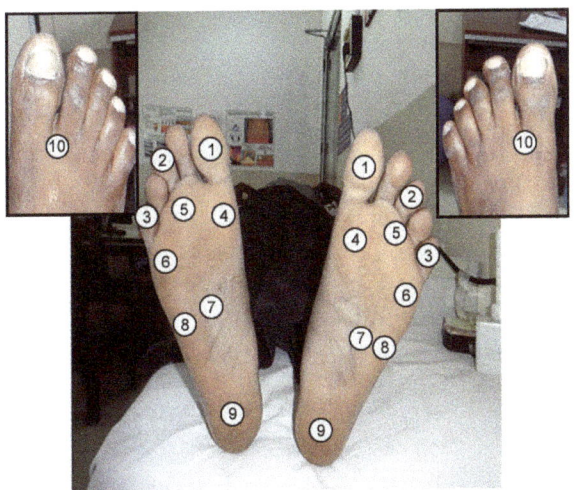

FIG. 5: The 10 sites for testing pressure sensation.

However, according to the International Working Group on the Diabetic Foot (IWGDF)-2019, one should examine in three points in the plantar aspect of the foot for the detection of diabetic foot. Patient is considered having neuropathy if they are not able to perceive in less than two out of three sites. The sites that were advised to be examined are shown in **Figure 6**.

Risk Categorization

Based on the foot examination, we can determine the patient's risk (**Table 3**) (individuals who are identified as "increased/high risk" may require a more comprehensive examination).

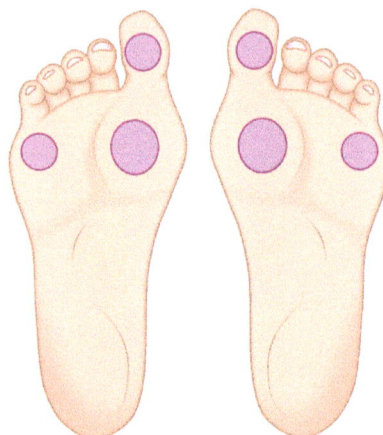

FIG. 6: Areas for the examination of monofilaments as per the International Working Group on the Diabetic Foot (IWGDF)-2019.

TABLE 3: Showing risk categorization of patients.

Risk category	Findings	Action
Low risk	Normal sensation and palpable pulses (All sites +ve)	Annual review and diabetes foot education
Increased risk	Neuropathy (>8 sites +ve) or absent pulses or other risk factors (poor footwear, social circumstances, poor diabetes control)	Refer to podiatry and diabetes foot education
High risk	Neuropathy (<8 sites +ve) or absent pulses plus foot deformity or skin changes/thickening (erythema, callous/corn previous ulcer or amputation)	Refer to podiatry and diabetes foot education
Emergency	New ulceration, swelling spreading cellulitis discoloration	Follow acute diabetic foot pathway

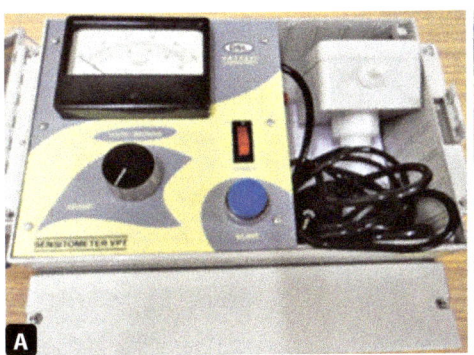 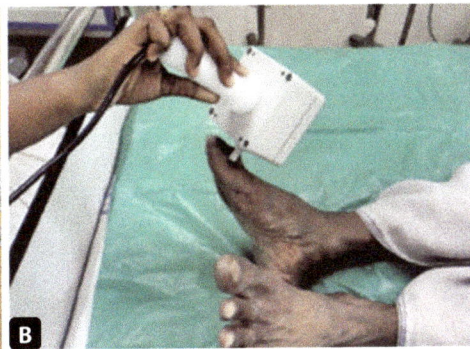

FIGS. 7A AND B: Biothesiometer.

Vibration Perception Threshold Measurement

Vibration perception may be assessed by a 128 Hz tuning fork. Vibration threshold measurements can be objectively done using an instrument called a biothesiometer. The biothesiometer is nothing but a tuning fork with graded vibration that gives a quantification of the vibration perception up to a maximum of 50 mV.

Neuropathy is considered to be present when a patient with DM cannot perceive >15 mV. It may be graded as mild—15–25 mV, moderate—25–40 mV, and severe >40 mV. In patients who are beyond the age of 70 years, one should consider neuropathy, when the patient cannot perceive >25 mV (**Figs. 7A** and **B**).

Nerve Conduction Studies

Electromyography-nerve conduction velocity (EMG-NCV) has emerged as an important method in tracing early onset and progression of peripheral neuropathy. They are objective, parametric, noninvasive, and sensitive measures. The main role of the EMG is to differentiate diabetic neuropathy from neuropathy of non-diabetic origin. Studies have mentioned that a significant reduction of NCV was observed in patients with mean HbA1c >10% over a period of 8 years.

NEWER TECHNIQUES

Newer techniques for evaluating small-fiber function include the use of:
- Corneal confocal microscopy, which allows the identification of unmyelinated axons in the cornea
- Sudomotor function devices

The algorithm for diagnostic evaluation of a patient suspected to have DM is shown in **Flowchart 2**.

Peripheral Neuropathy: Clinical Approach

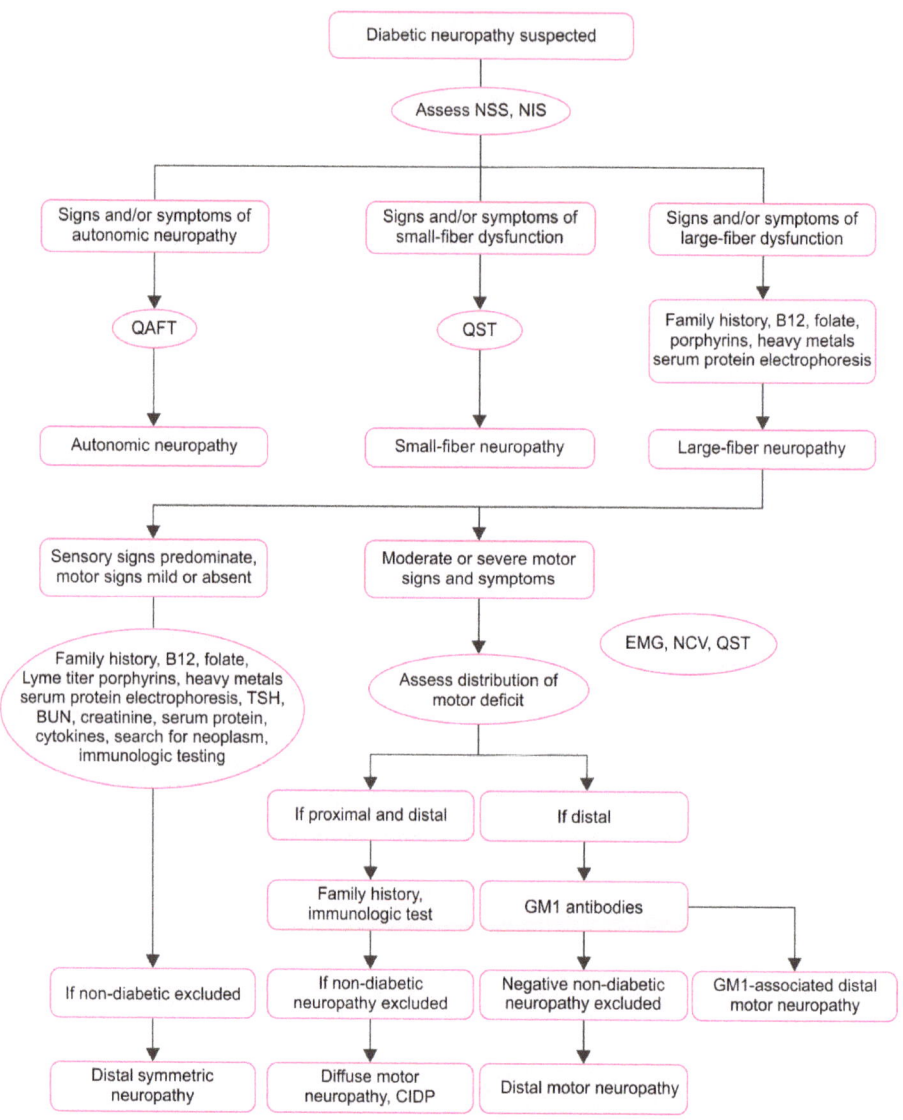

[B12: vitamin B12; BUN: blood urea nitrogen; CIDP: chronic inflammatory demyelinating polyneuropathy; EMG: electromyogram; GM1 antibodies: ganglioside GM1 antibodies; NCV: nerve conduction velocity studies; NIS: neurologic impairment score (sensory and motor evaluation); NSS: neurologic symptoms score; QAFT: quantitative autonomic function tests; QST: quantitative sensory tests; TSH: thyroid-stimulating hormone]

FLOWCHART 2: Stepwise investigation of a patient suspected to have diabetic neuropathy.

Source: Adapted from Medscape; endocrine practice, 2007 American Association of Clinical Endocrinologists.

TREATMENT

General Management

Small Fiber Neuropathy

- Daily foot inspection
- A hand held mirror to inspect the soles of the feet
- Microcellular rubber (MCR) shoes should fit well.
- Avoid exposure to extreme temperatures
- Moisturizing creams for skin drying and cracking
- After bathing, feet should be dried.
- Nails should be cut transversely.

Large Fiber Neuropathy

- *Gait and strength training*: Patients with DM and large-fiber neuropathy have an increased propensity to falls due to sensory ataxia, incoordination, weakness, muscle wasting, and resultant fracture following a fall, especially in the post-menopausal women. Hence, improving muscle strength is important in preventing complications related to DM and large-fiber neuropathy.
- MCR footwear (**Fig. 7A**)

Microcellular rubber is the most common material used in patients with DM and peripheral neuropathy. A shore value between 8 and 15 is ideal for footwear that is prescribed for those with DM. MCR footwear gives satisfactory results in preventing ulcer development as well as recurrence.

TREATMENT OF PAINFUL DIABETIC NEUROPATHY

Painful diabetic neuropathy (PDN) is a challenging problem for the treating physician. Controlling the blood glucose control is the first line of management in these patients. More often, simple analgesic therapy may not be sufficient enough to fully alleviate the symptoms. There are multiple pharmacological and nonpharmacological options for management of PDN. Patients should be offered various therapeutic options in a stepwise fashion.

Symptomatic Pharmacological Treatment of Painful Diabetic Neuropathy

Tricyclic Antidepressants

Tricyclic antidepressants are one of the most extensively used medication for the management of PDN. They reduce the pain sensation by multiple mechanisms. They act by inhibition of norepinephrine and/or serotonin reuptake at synapses of central descending pain control pathway and antagonizing N-methyl-D-aspartate receptor which mediates hyperalgesia. Some agents such as amitriptyline have additional sodium-channel blocking effect also.

Amitriptyline, imipramine, desipramine, and nortriptyline have shown efficacy in various studies. The number needed to treat (NNT) for >50% pain relief for amitriptyline is 2.4 (2.0–3.0). The initial dose is 10 mg once daily at night, to increase the dose by 25 mg at a time to reach a maximum tolerated dose of up to 150 mg/day. The most frequent side effects noted with TCAs are dry mouth, increased daytime somnolence, and tiredness. The number needed to harm for major adverse events was 19. It should be used with caution in patients with postural hypotension, recent myocardial infarction, especially with cardiac conduction blocks, decompensated heart failure, history of cardiac arrhythmias, presence of a long QT syndrome, bladder outlet obstruction, as well as angle-closure glaucoma.

Selective Serotonin Reuptake Inhibitors

As the name indicates, these medications selectively inhibit the presynaptic reuptake of serotonin thus decreasing the pain sensation. Agents such as paroxetine and citalopram showed significant pain relief in various studies, although less effective than TCAs. For selective serotonin reuptake inhibitors (SSRI), overall NNT is 7. Paroxetine was used as a fixed daily dose of 40 mg. The maximum efficacy is obtained with a blood level of 300–400 nmol/L. The side effect profile of SSRI is better than TCAs. There was increased risk of upper gastrointestinal bleeding documented in one randomized controlled trial (RCT). The risk increases if they are combined with nonsteroidal anti-inflammatory drugs (NSAIDs).

Serotonin Norepinephrine Reuptake Inhibitors

Serotonin norepinephrine reuptake inhibitors (SNRIs) act by dual selective inhibition of serotonin and norepinephrine. Duloxetine and venlafaxine are the medications in this class. Duloxetine was the first medication approved by the United States Food and Drug Administration (US FDA) for the treatment of PDN in 2004.

The initial dose of duloxetine is 30 mg/day for initial 4–5 days. Duloxetine at the dose of 60 mg/day and 120 mg/day are shown to be effective in pain reduction. The NNT for duloxetine is 4.9 for 120 mg/day and 5.2 for 60 mg/day. The numbers needed to harm based on discontinuation rates were 8.8 and 17.5 for 120 mg/day and 60 mg/day, respectively. The initial venlafaxine dosage is 75 mg/day and a maximum dose of 225 mg/day was also shown to significantly reduce the pain with a NNT of 6.9.

The major adverse events noted with 120 mg/day of duloxetine include nausea (27%), somnolence (28%), dizziness (23%), constipation (10%), and dry mouth (15%).

Calcium-channel Modulators [Alpha 2-delta ($\alpha 2\delta$) Ligands]

Gabapentin is one of the anticonvulsants related to gamma aminobutyric acid used in the treatment of PDN. This medication acts by binding to the $\alpha 2\delta$ subunit of voltage-activated calcium channels and inhibiting the channels, thus reducing excitatory neurotransmitter release. The initial dosage of gabapentin is 300 mg/day and the maximum dose tolerated is 3,600 mg/day. The NNT for >50% pain reduction was documented to be 3.7. In general, gabapentin is well-tolerated, however, dizziness and somnolence are the most frequent dose-dependent adverse events noted, affecting up to 23% of patients.

Pregabalin is approved by the US FDA for the treatment of PDN. Pregabalin is a more specific inhibitor of α2δ subunit of voltage-gated calcium channels. The starting dose is 50 mg/day and the maximum tolerated dose is 600 mg/day. The NNT for >50% pain reduction documented to be 4 (600 mg/day), 5.9 (300 mg/day), and 20 (150 mg/day). The adverse events noted with pregabalin are dizziness (22%), somnolence (12%), peripheral edema (10%), head ache (7%), and weight gain (5%).

Sodium-channel Blockers

There are multiple anticonvulsant medications were tried in the treatment of PDN such as sodium valproate, carbamazepine, oxcarbamazepine, lamotrigine, topiramate, and lacosamide. Sodium valproate is shown to be effective in PDN. Carbamazepine has only limited data available for treatment of PDN and was used extensively in the past. Lacosamide and lamotrigine are undergoing clinical trials for treatment of PDN. A randomized double-blinded study in 59 patients supported the use of lamotrigine as compared to placebo at different doses (200, 300, and 400 mg/day).

Opioids

Tramadol is a widely used opioid analgesic agent with a lower risk of development of tolerance and dependence. Nevertheless, dependence can certainly occur. This medication acts via opioids receptors and indirectly via monoaminergic receptor system. The initial dose is 50 mg/day and maximum tolerated dose is 400 mg/day. The NNT is documented to be 3.8. The most frequently noted adverse events include nausea (23%), constipation (21%), and headache (17%).

Oxycodone is a strong opioid analgesic used in more severe cases of PDN. Oxycodone is a pure μ agonist with a potent analgesic effect. Starting dose is 10 mg/day and maximum tolerated dose is 100 mg/day.

Other opioid analgesics such as morphine and tapentadol extended release were tried in treatment of PDN in short duration and small sample-sized studies. A combination of morphine and gabapentin showed better efficacy as compared to monotherapy.

Topical Agents

Capsaicin

Capsaicin (trans-8-methyl-N-vanillyl-6-nonenamide), an astringent, is an alkaloid with analgesic property. Substance P which is considered as the primary neurotransmitter of painful stimuli is depleted by capsaicin. Several studies have documented significant pain reduction and quality of life improvement with topical capsaicin therapy. The NNT for capsaicin cream (0.075%) is 5.7. The side effects of capsaicin therapy include burning sensation (60%), skin irritation (6.5%), erythema (7.2%) and dry skin (3.6%).

Topical nitrates and topical TCA doxepin are shown to be effective in PDN but with variable positive effects.

Nonpharmacologic Measures for Treatment of Painful Diabetic Neuropathy

There are a number of nonpharmacologic treatment modalities for PDN. They are often used in patients with severe pain not controlled with multiple pharmacologic measures.

Transcutaneous Electrical Nerve Stimulation

This is a method by which electrical stimuli of various frequencies and intensities are applied to the skin surface for various duration, resulting in pain relief. This technique is used for different acute and chronic pain conditions.

The transcutaneous electrical nerve stimulation (TENS) application can either be low frequency (<10 Hz) or high frequency (50–100 Hz and above). TENS causes analgesia by multiple mechanisms at the peripheral, spinal, and supraspinal levels. At the periphery, it was demonstrated to decrease the effect of serotonin in pain perception. By stimulating the Aβ afferent fibers, it inhibits the nociceptive activity at the dorsal horn of spinal cord. However, RCTs of TENS failed to show a significant reduction in symptomatic PDN.

Frequency-modulated Electromagnetic Nerve Stimulation

Frequency-modulated electromagnetic nerve stimulation (FREMS) uses sequences of modulated electrical stimuli that vary in their pulse frequency, duration, and voltage amplitude automatically. Summation of subthreshold stimuli result in inducing composite motor action potential in excitable tissue. In a randomized controlled study, it showed a significant reduction in day time and nighttime pain scores.

Electrical Spinal Cord Stimulation

Electrical spinal cord stimulation (ESCS) have been used for various acute and chronic pain conditions. Electrical stimuli are given via ESCS electrode inserted to the epidural space. In a small numbered placebo-controlled trial, 8 out of 10 patients showed 50% reduction in pain score immediately after the procedure. At the end of 14 months, 6 patients were having significant pain relief without any other agents for analgesia.

Treatment of PDN is based on following pathogenic concepts:
- *Glycemic control*: Data from the Diabetes Control and Complications Trial (DCCT) suggested that intensive glucose control resulted in primary and secondary prevention of peripheral neuropathy in patients with Type 1 diabetes mellitus. Overall, it reduced the occurrence of clinical neuropathy by 60%.
- *Alpha-lipoic acid (ALA)*: ALA is an antioxidant which helps in reducing the oxidative stress thus causing symptom relief in patients with distal sensory neuropathy. Long-term placebo-controlled trials have failed to demonstrate a clinically significant pain reduction in patients.

- *Aldose reductase inhibitor (ARI)*: By blocking the polyol pathway, ARIs have been proposed to reverse the peripheral neuropathy in patients with diabetes mellitus. Early trials of most of the ARIs showed significant side effects with limited efficacy. Epalristat had shown improvement in patient reported neuropathic symptoms with a favorable side effect profile but needs large-scale randomized trial to prove its efficacy.
- *Other agents*: Medications such as benfotiamine and protein kinase C inhibitor (ruboxistaurin) failed to show clinically significant symptom relief in long-term trials of patients with diabetes mellitus and peripheral neuropathy.

TREATMENT OF DIABETIC AMYOTROPHY

Diabetic amyotrophy is a distinct entity with varied presentation. Moreover, it would be oversimplification to ascribe amyotrophy simply due to DM, as many other causative factors are associated with this presentation. Moreover, specific treatment modalities directed at individual causes can have dramatic response. Diabetic amyotrophy almost always coexists with diabetic sensorimotor polyneuropathy (DSPN). EMG reveals lumbosacral plexopathy. If demyelination predominates in EMG, a diagnosis of CIDP, MGUS, or vasculitis should be kept as a differential diagnosis. The treatment for the above-mentioned disorders is with steroid and immunosuppressants.

With Reference to the Aforementioned Patient 1

His serum vitamin B12, folic acid, and electrophoresis were normal. His work-up for secondary causes of peripheral neuropathy was negative. His EMG also showed axonal neuropathy with involvement to suggest demyelination. There was no significant improvement in his sensory symptoms in spite of initiating amitriptyline at a dose of 75 mg/day. The dose of pregabalin and amitriptyline was not further increased as he developed lethargy which was hampering his daily activities. As the patient was already on optimal medical therapy without much benefit, he was advised TENS. The patient was better after the treatment with multiple sessions of TENS therapy.

For the second patient, he was investigated further in view of the discordance between the duration of diabetes and absence of other microvascular complications of diabetes except for severe neuropathy. His investigations were negative for multiple myeloma. Nerve conduction study done showed demyelinating polyneuropathy. Positron emission tomography (PET) scan done to rule out any occult malignancy was negative. Hence, a diagnosis of CIDP was made. The patient was treated with intravenous immunoglobulin and has been on follow-up.

CONCLUSION

Peripheral neuropathy is the most common complication of DM. It is important to rule out other secondary causes of neuropathy before labeling it as a diabetes-related peripheral neuropathy.

Management of patients with diabetic neuropathy includes medical therapy for neuropathy, blood glucose management, and newer therapy which includes, TENS, electrical spinal cord stimulation (SCS), and percutaneous electrical nerve stimulation (PENS) may be used in those with refractory painful neuropathy.

REFERENCES

1. Armstrong DG, Lavery LA, Harkless LB. Validation of a diabetic wound classification system. The contribution of depth, infection, and ischemia to risk of amputation. Diabetes Care. 1998;21(5):855-9.
2. Consensus statement: Report and recommendations of the San Antonio conference on diabetic neuropathy. American Diabetes Association American Academy of Neurology. Diabetes Care. 1988;11(7):592-7.
3. Casellini C, Vinik A. Clinical manifestations and current treatment options for diabetic neuropathies. Endocr Pract. 2007;13(5):550-66.
4. Bansal D, Gudala K, Muthyala H, Esam HP, Nayakallu R, Bhansali A. Prevalence and risk factors of development of peripheral diabetic neuropathy in type 2 diabetes mellitus in a tertiary care setting. J Diabetes Investig. 2014;5(6):714-21.
5. Sugimoto K, Nishizawa Y, Horiuchi S, Yagihashi S. Localization in human diabetic peripheral nerve of N(epsilon)-carboxymethyllysine-protein adducts, an advanced glycation endproduct. Diabetologia. 1997;40(12):1380-7.
6. Sander HW, Chokroverty S. Diabetic amyotrophy: current concepts. Semin Neurol. 1996;16(2):173-8.
7. Yagihashi S, Mizukami H, Sugimoto K. Mechanism of diabetic neuropathy: Where are we now and where to go? J Diabetes Investig. 2011;2(1):18-32.

CHAPTER 4

MARCHAL de CALVI AND THOMAS HODGKIN

Marchal de Calvi in 1852 and Thomas Hodgkin in 1854, respectively, realized that there was an association between diabetes and gangrene of the foot. At that time, it was common to treat ulcers by prolonged bed rest, although it was noticed that the wounds would return once the patient was mobile again. A potential infection of foot ulcers could be a significant cause of morbidity and mortality in the 1850s, and hence the contribution of both Hodgkin and de Calvi was a significant advancement in the field. Hodgkin is also known for having described Hodgkin's Disease, a type of lymphoma, in 1832.

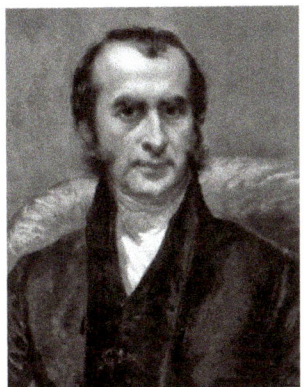

Thomas Hodgkin

Diabetic Foot Ulcers: Clinical Approach

Jinson Paul, Felix Jebasingh K, Kripa Elizabeth Cherian, Anand John Samuel G, Ruth Volena D, Nihal Thomas

CASE SCENARIOS

A 54-year-old lady with a history of diabetes mellitus (DM) for 15 years presented with high-grade fever, redness, and swelling of the left foot with an ulcer on the lateral aspect for 7 days. There was active discharge from the wound which was foul-smelling. She had undergone amputation of the left great toe 4 years before. On examination, her vital signs were stable, she was febrile, the left foot examination revealed erythema up to the ankle with induration, and mottling seen on the fourth and fifth toes. There was a deep ulcer of 2 × 2 cm over the webspace between the fourth and fifth toes. Bilateral peripheral pulses were well felt. The left inguinal lymph nodes were enlarged and tender. On further evaluation, she had bilateral distal symmetrical peripheral neuropathy, bilateral moderate nonproliferative diabetic retinopathy, and microalbuminuria. Her investigations revealed a random blood glucose level of 303 mg/dL, normocytic anemia, and neutrophilic leukocytosis. An X-ray of the left foot was normal. The patient was given empirical intravenous antibiotics. The patient underwent a transmetatarsal amputation of the left foot. She was discharged after 4 days and was regularly followed up with daily dressings at home (**Figs. 1A** to **C**).

INTRODUCTION

Diabetic foot ulcers (DFUs) are frequently encountered in patients with DM. Nearly 25% of patients with DM are affected by foot ulcers during their lifetime, with a population-based annual incidence (in the United States of America) between 1 and 4.1%.[1] Diabetes remains the most common cause of nontraumatic amputation worldwide with a 15 times higher incidence than those without diabetes. Over 85% of lower limb amputations are preceded by foot ulcers.[2] A multicentric study done in four different centers in India found that the prevalence of diabetic foot infection was 6–11% and the prevalence of amputation was 3%.[3] Diabetic foot complications remain major medical, social, and economic problems across the world. According

Diabetic Foot Ulcers: Clinical Approach

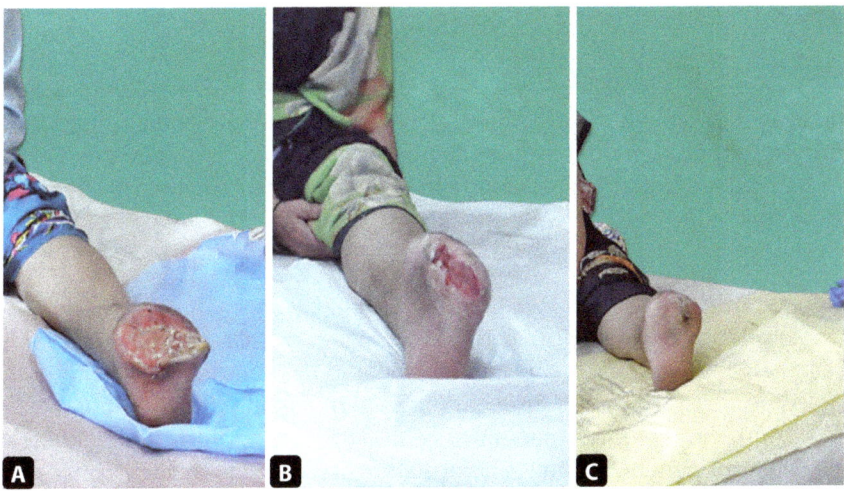

FIGS. 1A TO C: Serial pictures of the foot ulcer (post-trans-metatarsal amputation) with time frame. (A) During the first visit; (B) After 6 months; (C) After 15 months.

to the 2007 data from the United States of America, $18.9 billion (1,800 crore in INR) was spent on the care of DFUs and $11.7 billion (800 crore in INR) on lower extremity amputations. Diabetes-related foot ulcer causes debilitating effects in the social, economic, and psychological aspects both among the patients and the caretakers. Most often the diabetes foot ulcer is preventable. Unfortunately, many patients due to lack of availability of adequate care tend to get delayed treatment and thereby end up with minor to major lower limb amputations.

One should keep involvement of mind the importance of salvaging the affected limb as well as the prevention of the involvement of the contralateral limb which is also at risk for acquiring a foot ulcer. Studies have proven that a patient with an amputation in one limb, has 10–20 times greater risk of amputation of any kind on the contralateral limb over a follow-up period of 3 years. In other words, half of patients will have another amputation within the first 5 years of an amputation. It is only possible by recognizing the factors that negatively influence the prognosis that the number of amputations can be reduced. It imposes a major economic burden to the individual and the society.[4]

The tragic rule of 15:
- 15–25% of people with diabetes will develop a foot ulcer in their lifetime.
- 15% of foot ulcers will develop osteomyelitis.
- 15% of foot ulcers will lead to an amputation.

Tragic rule of 50:
- 50% of amputations are at a trans-femoral/trans-tibial level.[5,6]
- 50% of patients need second amputation in 5 years.
- 50% of patients die at 5 years.[7,8]

ETIOLOGY AND CLASSIFICATION OF DIABETIC FOOT ULCERS

Diabetic foot ulcers can be of three types—neuropathic, ischemic, and neuroischemic. Neuropathy, peripheral vascular disease, and increased foot pressure are the major pathogenic factors for development of the DFU. Pathogenesis of DFU is shown in **Flowchart 1**.

Neuropathic Ulcers

Neuropathy is associated with an 8- to 10-fold higher risk of ulceration and 2- to 5-fold higher risk of amputation. The mechanism behind the neuropathic ulcer is complex. First, it is because of a loss of protective sensation leading to reduced perception of pain. Second, the motor component of neuropathy causes intrinsic weakness of the muscular compartment, leading to deformation of toe flexion (mainly by interosseous and lumbricals), which results in formation of overloaded plantar areas. The intrinsic muscles of the foot are shown in **Figure 2**. Moreover, the autonomic dysfunction causes anhidrosis and thereby dry skin and arteriovenous (AV) shunting, leading on to alteration of blood supply to the skin and underlying bones.

Neuropathic ulcers usually occur on the plantar aspect of the foot most commonly under the first metatarsal head and tip of the toes (**Figs. 3A** to **C**). The most common cause of ulceration is due to the abnormal pressure distribution and consequent repetitive mechanical forces of gait and the resultant callus formation. Untreated callosity is a preulcerative lesion in the diabetic neuropathic foot (**Flowchart 2**).

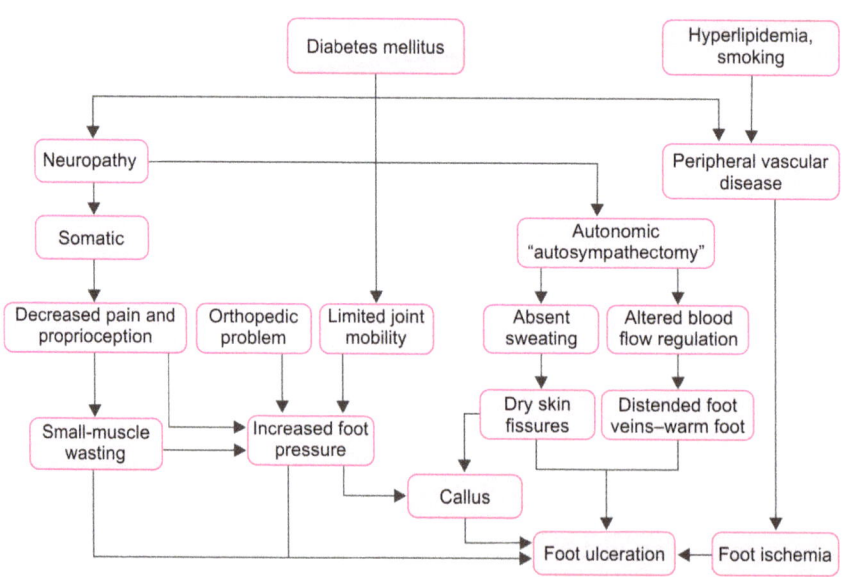

FLOWCHART 1: Pathogenesis of diabetic foot ulcer.

Diabetic Foot Ulcers: Clinical Approach

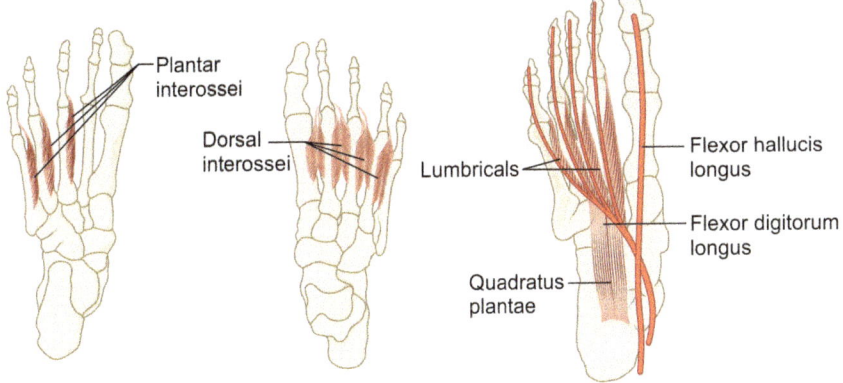

FIG. 2: Showing muscles of foot.

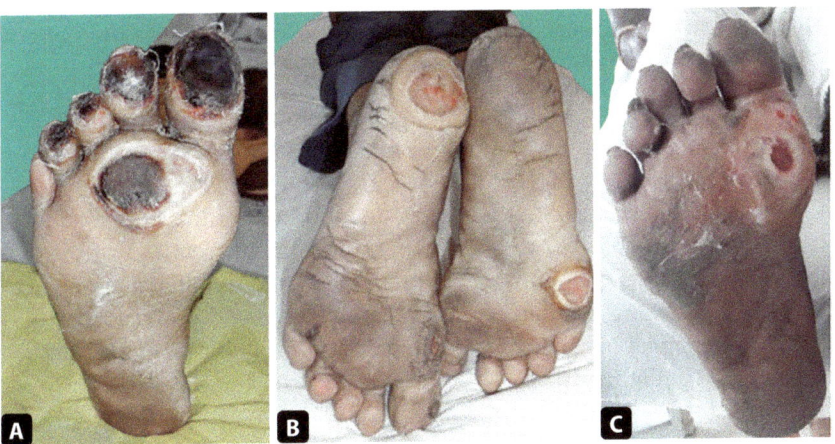

FIGS. 3A TO C: Showing sites of neuropathic ulcers—(A) Over plantar aspects of the toes, (B) Heel and fifth metatarsal head, and (C) First metatarsal head.

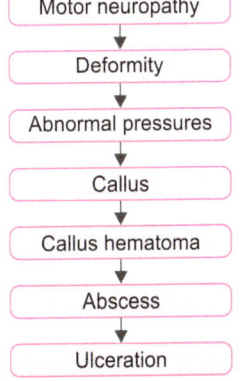

FLOWCHART 2: Mechanism of callosity developing to ulcer.

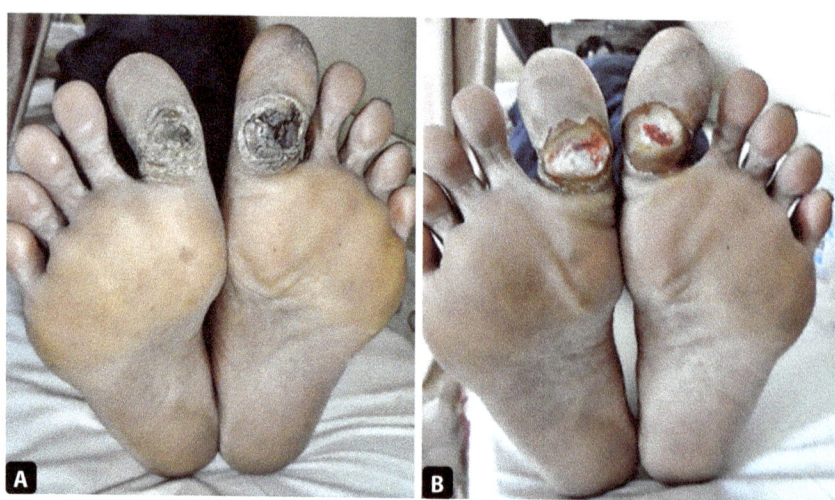

FIGS. 4A AND B: Showing—(A) Callosities present over the plantar aspects of both great toes, and (B) The underlying ulcer exposed on removal of the callosities.

Therefore, thick callus may press on the soft tissues beneath and cause ulceration (**Figs. 4A** and **B**).

A layer of whitish, macerated, moist tissue found under the surface of the callus indicates that the foot is close to ulceration, and urgent removal of the callus is required. If the callus is not removed, inflammatory autolysis and hematomas develop under the callus leading to tissue necrosis, resulting in a small cavity filled with serous fluid giving the appearance of a blister under the callus. Removal of the callus reveals an ulcer as seen in **Figure 4B**.

Ischemic and Neuroischemic Ulcers

Ischemic and neuroischemic ulcers are commonly located at the margins of the foot, often on the medial surface of the first and over the lateral aspect of the fifth metatarsophalangeal joint. In addition, they develop on the tips of the toes and beneath toe nails if these become overtly thick (**Figs. 5A** and **B**). The classic signs of preulceration in the neuroischemic foot are a red mark on the skin, often tight shoes due to small-sized shoe, leading to frictional forces on the vulnerable margins of the foot. The features of neuropathic, ischemic, and neuroischemic ulcers are shown in **Table 1**.

The cardinal sign of ischemic ulceration is a superficial blister, following persistent friction that develops into a shallow ulcer with a base of sparse pale granulation tissue or yellowish closely adherent slough. There can be associated features such as brittle nails and the absence of hair.

Despite delivering exemplary wound care, wounds may fail to heal due to a variety of reasons such as poor glycemic control, lack of blood flow, unrelieved pressure, poor care, infection, and coexisting systemic diseases.

Diabetic Foot Ulcers: Clinical Approach

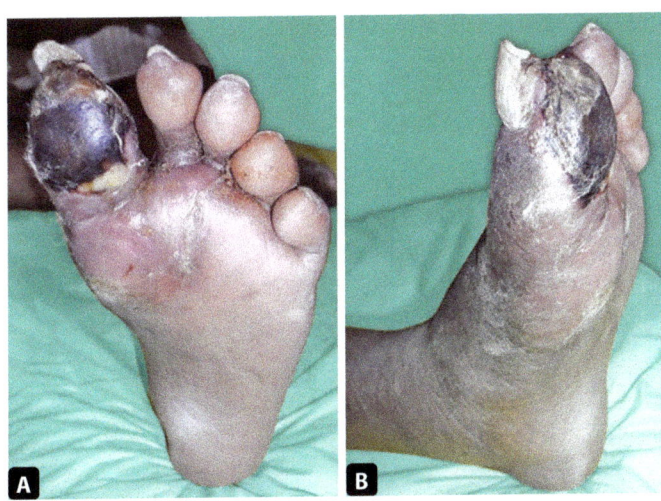

FIGS. 5A AND B: A neuroischemic ulcer over the great toe.

TABLE 1: Features of neuropathic and ischemic ulcers.

Features	Neuropathic	Ischemic	Neuroischemic
Sensation	Usually painless	Painful	Degree of sensory loss
Callus/necrosis	Callus present and often thick	Necrosis common	Minimal callus prone to necrosis
Wound bed	Pink and granulating, surrounded by callus	Pale and sloughy with poor granulation	Poor granulation
Foot temperature and pulses	Warm with bounding pulses	Cool and absent pulses	Cool with absent pulses
Other	Dry skin and fissuring	Delayed healing	High risk of infection
Typical location	Weight-bearing areas of the foot such as metatarsal heads, the heel and over the dorsum of clawed toes	Tips of toes, nail edges and between the toes and lateral borders of the foot	Margins of the foot and toes
Prevalence	35%	15%	50%

Infected Ulcers

Individuals with DM have increased risk of hospitalization with soft tissue and bone infections of the foot compared to those without DM.[9] Following are the factors that predispose the ulcer for an infection:
- Chronic poor glycemic control
- A positive probe-to-bone (PTB) test
- Ulcer for >30 days

Diabetic Foot Ulcers: Clinical Approach

TABLE 2: Modified Dundee classification of cellulitis.

Modified "Dundee" classification	
Class I	No sepsis, no comorbidities, and SEWS [Standardized Early Warning Score (**Table 3**)] <4
Class II	Documentation of one or more significant comorbidities (e.g., obesity, peripheral vascular disease or venous insufficiency), no sepsis, and SEWS <4
Class III	Sepsis but SEWS <4
Class IV	Sepsis and SEWS ≥4

Source: Clinical Resource Efficiency Support Team (CREST). Guidelines on the Management of Cellulitis in Adults. 2005.

TABLE 3: SEWS (Standardized Early Warning Score) parameters and scoring systems.

Parameter	Score						
	3	2	1	0	1	2	3
Respiratory rate (breaths/min)	≤8			9–20	21–30	31–35	≥36
Oxygen saturation (%)	<85	85–89	90–92	≥93			
Temperature (°C)	<34	34–34.9	35–35.9	36–37.9	38–38.4	≥38.5	
Systolic blood pressure (mm Hg)	≤69	70–79	80–99	100–199		≥200	
Heart rate (bpm)	≤29	30–39	40–49	50–99	100–109	110–129	≥130
AVPU response (stimulus required to induce response)	Unresponsive	Pain	Verbal	Alert			

[AVPU: alert, verbal, pain, unresponsive (category of stimulus required to generate patient response)]

Source: SEWS Chart. [online] Available from: www.nhslothian.scot.nhs.uk/health_promotion/sewskey.pdf. [Last accessed November, 2021].

- Recurrent foot ulcers
- Ulcer following a trauma
- Underlying peripheral vascular disease
- Past history of lower extremity amputation
- Loss of protective sensation (LOPS)
- Associated renal insufficiency
- Behaviors such as walking barefoot
- Cigarette smoking

The modified Dundee classification of a patient with cellulitis is shown in **Table 2**. As per the International Working Group on Diabetic Foot (IWGDF) recommendations, the clinicians should evaluate a patient with an ulcer: The affected foot or limb and

Diabetic Foot Ulcers: Clinical Approach

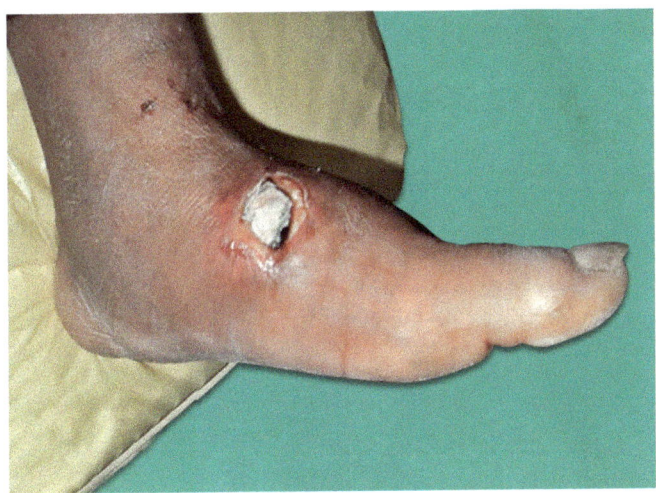

FIG. 6: Showing ulcer over the medial aspect of the foot with redness and swelling suggestive of underlying infection and cellulitis.

the infected wound as well as the opposite limb. Clinicians should diligently look for the presence of symptoms or signs of inflammation (erythema, warmth, tenderness, pain, or induration) or purulent secretions (**Fig. 6**). One should also look for arterial and venous insufficiency, LOPS, and biomechanical problem. Subsequently, the severity of the infection should be determined depending on its extent and depth and the presence of any systemic findings of infection. It is recommended to debride any wound that has necrotic tissue or a surrounding callus; the required procedure may range from minor to extensive.

AN APPROACH TO A FOOT ULCER

The approach to a foot ulcer should target various levels, such as systemic signs, neurological, vascular, dermatological, musculoskeletal, radiological, and at the laboratory. Other factors such as socioeconomic status, psychosocial influence, and diabetes-related complications should also be considered.

Foot examination should include assessment of skin temperature since increased warmth is the first indicator of inflammation in the insensate foot. Skin color, thickness, dryness, cracking, perspiration, webspace infection, ulceration, calluses, blistering, hemorrhage, etc., should be observed while inspecting a diabetic foot. Deformities such as claw toes, hammer toe, mallet toe, bunion (**Figs. 7A** and **B**), prominent metatarsal heads, muscle wasting (guttering between metatarsals), and Charcot foot (**Fig. 7C**) should also be looked for in the foot.[10] The loss of sensation over the distal plantar surface to the 10 g Semmes Weinstein monofilament (5.08 g) is a significant and independent predictor of future foot ulceration and the possibility of lower-extremity amputation.

Diabetic Foot Ulcers: Clinical Approach

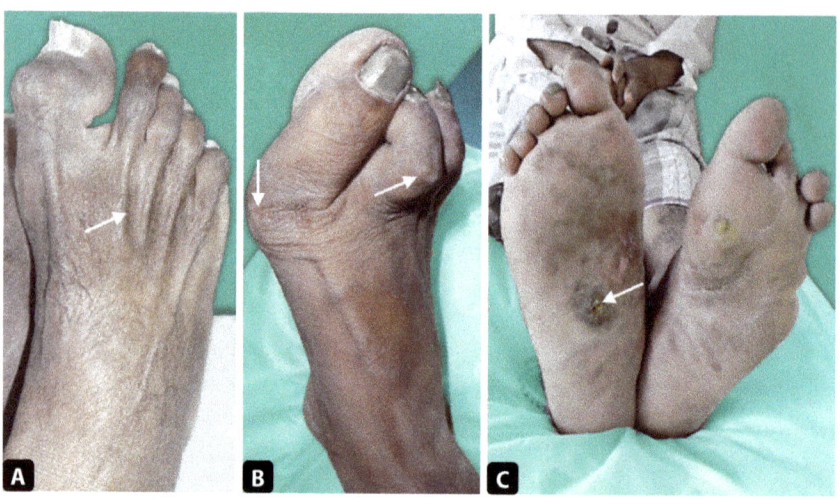

FIGS. 7A TO C: (A) Claw toe, (B) Bunion and hammer toes, and (C) Charcot foot with ulcer.

TABLE 4: The Society for Vascular Technology's interpretation of resting ABPI measurements.

Resting ABPI	Severity of disease
>1.4	Calcification may be present
>1.0	Probably no arterial disease
0.81–1.00	No significant arterial disease, or mild/insignificant disease
0.5–0.80	Moderate disease
<0.5	Severe disease
<0.4	Critical ischemia

(ABPI: ankle brachial pressure index)
Source: Al-Qaisi M, Nott DM, King DH, Kaddoura S. Ankle brachial pressure index (ABPI): An update for practitioners. Vasc Health Risk Manag. 2009;5:833-41.

In persons with DM and underlying ischemia, the distribution of peripheral arterial disease (PAD) is greater in the arteries below the knee. Simple bedside evaluation for PAD includes noninvasive assessments such as ankle brachial blood pressure index (ABPI), determination of systolic toe pressure by photoplethysmography (PPG), transcutaneous oximetry (TcPO$_2$), and Doppler arterial flow studies.

Although the ABPI is an easy and reliable tool, many a time it underestimates the degree of peripheral arterial occlusive disease (PAOD) amongst those with arterial calcification (**Table 4**).

Moreover, ulcers occur on the plantar surface of the foot in areas with increased pressure, due to the excessive repetitive and shear force. Almost half of the patients present with recurrent ulcer, either at the same foot or in the opposite foot if not intervened with appropriate footwear after the initial ulcer heals.

Diabetic Foot Ulcers: Clinical Approach

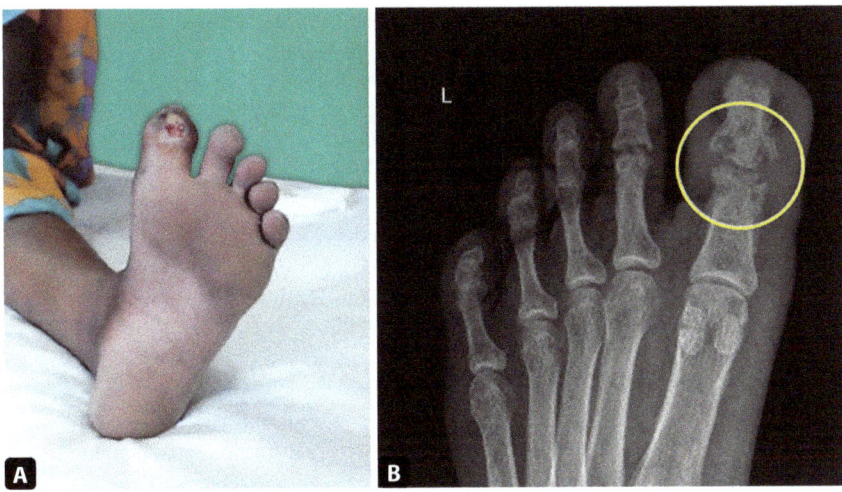

FIGS. 8A AND B: (A) An ulcer over the great toe with probe test being negative and (B) X-ray of the same patient showing osteomyelitis of the proximal and distal phalanges of the left great toe (Shown with a circle).

The most common site of ulcer is the base of the first metatarsal bone followed by the apex of the toes, bases of other metatarsals, and mid-foot ulcers.

Assessment of bone involvement is an important factor as it determines the ulcer healing. This has been explained in greater detail in the chapter on osteomyelitis. The involvement of the phalanges of left great toe with an ulcer is shown in **Figures 8A** and **B**.

Classification of Foot Ulcers

There are various classification systems which have been proposed (**Table 5**), most commonly cited ones are mentioned here.

The key features of various classifications are as follows:
- Classification systems grade ulcers according to the presence and extent of various physical characteristics, such as size, depth, appearance, and location.
- They can help in the planning and monitoring of treatment and in predicting outcome and can be used for research and audit.

Management of Foot Ulcers

Ulcer Dressing

Some studies show better healing rate with hydrogels in small ulcer comparing to gauze dressing. Whatever technique is used, achievement of the following goals is important in wound care:
- Promote granulation (new tissue containing all the cellular components for epithelialization)

Diabetic Foot Ulcers: Clinical Approach

TABLE 5: Key features of various classification systems for foot ulcers.

Classification system	Key points	Pros/Cons
Wagner (Table 8)	Assesses ulcer depth along with the presence of gangrene and the loss of perfusion using six grades (0–5)	• Well established • Does not fully address infection and ischemia
University of Texas (Table 6) (Armstrong)	Assesses ulcer depth, presence of infection and presence of the signs of lower-extremity ischemia using a matrix of four grades combined with four stages	• Well established • Describes the presence of infection and ischemia much better than the Wagner classification and may help in predicting the outcome of the DFU
PEDIS (Table 7) (PEDIS—perfusion, extent, depth, infection, and sensation)	Assesses Perfusion, Extent (size), Depth (tissue loss), Infection and Sensation (neuropathy) using four grades (1–4)	• Developed by IWGDF (International Working Group on Diabetic Foot) • User-friendly (clear definitions, few categories) for practitioners with a lower level of experience with diabetic foot management
SINBAD (Table 9) (site, ischemia, neuropathy, bacterial infection, area, and depth)	• Assesses site, ischemia, neuropathy, bacterial infection, and depth • Uses a scoring system to help predict outcomes and enable comparisons between different settings and countries	Simplified version of the S(AD) SAD classification system Includes ulcer site as data suggests this might be an important determinant of outcome

TABLE 6: University of Texas classification.

Stage	Grade			
	0	1	2	3
A (no infection or ischemia)	Pre- or post-ulcerative lesion completely epithelialized	Superficial wound not involving tendon capsule, or bone	Wound penetrating to tendon or capsule	Wound penetrating to bone or joint
B	Infection	Infection	Infection	Infection
C	Ischemia	Ischemia	Ischemia	Ischemia
D	Infection and ischemia	Infection and ischemia	Infection and ischemia	Infection and ischemia

Source: Armstrong DG, Lavery LA, Harkless LB. Validation of a diabetic wound classification system: the contribution of depth, infection and vascular disease to the risk of amputation. Diabetes Care. 1998;21(5): 855-9.

TABLE 7: PEDIS classification of severity of diabetic foot infections.

Clinical criteria	Grade/severity
No clinical signs of infection	Grade 1/uninfected
Superficial tissue lesion with at least two of the following signs: • Local warmth • Erythema >0.5–2 cm around the ulcer • Local tenderness/pain • Local swelling/induration • Purulent discharge Other causes of inflammation of the skin must be excluded	Grade 2/mild
Erythema >2 cm and one of the findings above or: • Infection involving structures beneath the skin/subcutaneous tissues (e.g., deep abscess, lymphangitis, osteomyelitis, septic arthritis, or fasciitis) • No systemic inflammatory response	Grade 3/moderate
Presence of systemic signs with at least two of the following: • Temperature >39°C or <36°C • Pulse >90 bpm • Respiratory rate >20/min • $PaCO_2$ <32 mm Hg • White cell count 12,000 mm^3 or <4,000 mm^3 • 10% immature leukocytes	Grade 4/severe

Source: Abbas Z, Lutale JK, Game FL, Jeffcoate WJ. Comparison of four systems of classification of diabetic foot ulcers in Tanzania. Diabet Med. 2008;25(2):134-7.

TABLE 8: Wagner–Meggitt classification.

Grades	Foot-related symptoms
Grade 1	Superficial ulcers
Grade 2	Deep ulcers
Grade 3	Ulcers with bone involvement
Grade 4	Partial gangrene
Grade 5	Complete gangrene

Source: Oyibo SO, Jude EB, Tarawneh I, Nguyen HC, Harkless LB, Boulton AJ. A comparison of two diabetic foot ulcer classification systems: the Wagner and the University of Texas wound classification systems. Diabetes care. 2001;24(1):84-8.

TABLE 9: SINBAD classification.

Category	Definition	Score
Site	• Forefoot	0
	• Midfoot	1
Ischemia	• Pedal pulses intact (at least one pulse palpable)	0
	• Clinical evidence of reduced pedal blood flow	1

Continued

Continued

Category	Definition	Score
Neuropathy	• Protective sensation intact	0
	• Protective sensation lost	1
Bacterial infection	• None	0
	• Present	1
Area	• Ulcer <1 cm²	0
	• Ulcer ≥1 cm²	1
Depth	• Ulcer confined to skin and subcutaneous tissue	0
	• Ulcer reaching muscle, tendon, or deeper	1
Total possible score		6

Source: Beckert S, Witte M, Wicke C, Königsrainer A, Coerper S. A new wound-based severity score for diabetic foot ulcers. Diabetes Care. 2006;29(5):988-92.

- Autolytic processes (wherein host-generated enzymes help break down devitalized tissues)
- Angiogenesis (new blood vessel formation)
- More rapid migration of epidermal cells across the wound base

The selection of wound dressings should be based on the wound bed characteristics:
- If dry, it should be hydrated.
- If draining, the exudate should be absorbed.
- If necrotic, it should be debrided.

Ideal characteristics of dressing are as follows:
- High moisture vapor permeability
- Nonadherent
- High capacity for absorption
- Provides barrier to external contaminants
- Prevents capillary loops penetrating into dressing material
- Good adhesion to the surrounding skin
- Hypoallergenic
- Comfortable
- Cost-effective

Negative Pressure Wound Therapy

Negative pressure wound therapy (NPWT) is a noninvasive wound closure system that uses controlled, localized negative pressure to help healing wounds.[11] This is explained in detail in the NPWT chapter.

Debridement

Debridement is the removal of necrotic and senescent tissues (**Fig. 9A**) or infected materials from a wound. This helps in reducing the local bacterial colonies, stimulation of the local growth factor, and proper facilitation of the wound drainage. In addition, maintaining the moisture in the wound is also important.

Diabetic Foot Ulcers: Clinical Approach

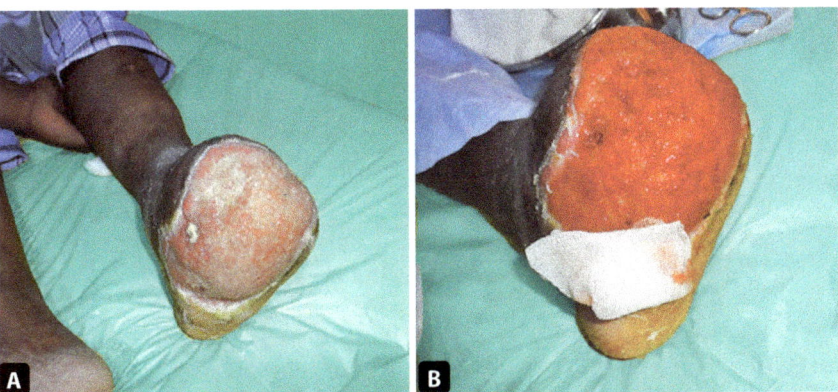

FIGS. 9A AND B: Showing a trans-metatarsal amputation stump ulcer (A) before and (B) after debridement of the slough.

The guiding principles for wound debridement are best remembered using the pneumonic, TIME:
- Tissue debridement
- Inflammation and infection control
- Moisture balance
- Epithelial edge advancement

There are many methods of debridement that are used in the management of DFUs including surgical/sharp, larval, autolytic, and, more recently, hydrosurgery and ultrasonic techniques. Debridement may be a one-off procedure or it may need to be ongoing for maintenance of the healthy wound bed (**Fig. 9B**). The requirement for further debridement should be determined at each dressing change.

Surgical Sharp Debridement

Sharp debridement is the gold standard technique for tissue management in DFUs which is regular, local, sharp debridement using a scalpel, scissors, and/or forceps. The benefits of sharp debridement are as follows:
- Removes necrotic/sloughy tissue
- Callus removal
- Reduces pressure
- Allows full inspection of the underlying tissues
- Helps drainage of secretions or pus
- Stimulates healing

Sharp debridement is recommended to remove all devitalized tissue or callus till the level of viable bleeding. It is important to debride the margins of the wound wherein the epithelium fails to be in level with the granulation base, so that the "edge effect" is prevented.

Sharp debridement is an invasive procedure. It is always important to probe the ulcer as this is a simple tool in diagnosing osteomyelitis. Moreover, if a subungual ulcer (**Figs. 10A** and **B**) is suspected, the nail should be cut straight or paired to drain the ulcer.

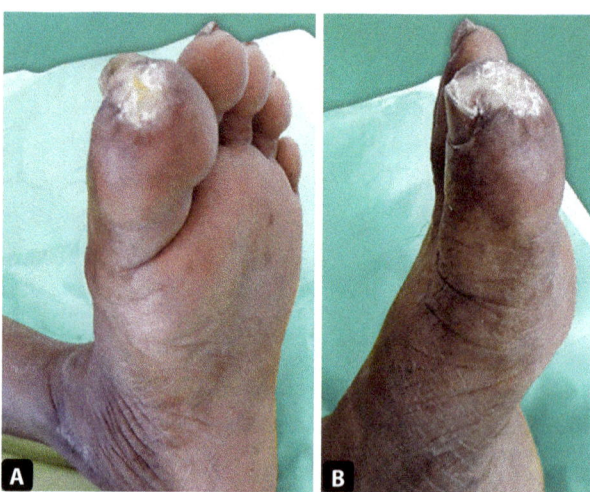

FIGS. 10A AND B: Subungual ulcer.

One should be aware that vascular status must always be determined prior to sharp debridement. Also, debridement should not be avoided in vascular compromised ulcers; a tooth-pick approach can be followed for removing the callus. However, the ideal time for debridement would be after revascularization.

Topical antimicrobials have no role in the treatment of DFU as there is little evidence over conventional saline dressing or dry dressing. The cost–benefit ratio is also high. One should also keep in mind that this unhealthy practice may cause bacterial resistance.

Microbiological Control

Most often patients with diabetes and foot ulcers can be managed in outpatient department (OPD). All ulcers need not be treated with antibiotics. Only if there is an evidence of severe infection, overlapped with an ischemic component, they may require admission. Patients with an infected ulcer or if in case there is a high risk for methicillin-resistant *Staphylococcus aureus* (MRSA) or *pseudomonas*, appropriate antibiotics should be initiated (**Table 10**).

Methicillin-resistant *Staphylococcus aureus* should be suspected when there is a previous history of hospitalization, previous wound infection with MRSA, an improperly treated previous infection, nasal carriage of MRSA, and evidence of osteomyelitis or a long-standing infection. Patients may be empirically treated for MRSA, if the infection is sufficiently severe.[12] The duration of treatment based on location, severity, extent of wound, and bone involvement is shown in **Table 11**.

Surgical indication for patients with diabetes and ulcer is discussed in the chapter on Surgeries in Diabetic Foot.

Diabetic foot ulcers should be managed in various levels such as wound control, microbiological control, metabolic control, mechanical control, and vascular control

Diabetic Foot Ulcers: Clinical Approach

TABLE 10: Suggested empirical antibiotic regimens based on clinical severity of diabetic foot infections.

Infection severity	Probable pathogen(s)	Antibiotic agent	Comments
Mild [usually treated with oral agent(s)]	*Staphylococcus aureus* (MSSA); *Streptococcus* species MRSA	• Clindamycin	• Requires QID dosing; narrow spectrum
		• Cephalexin	• Inexpensive, usually active against community-associated Methicillin-resistant *Staphylococcus aureus* (MRSA)
		• Levofloxacin	• Requires QID dosing; inexpensive
		• Amoxicillin-clavulanate	• Once-daily dosing; suboptimal against *S. aureus*
		• Doxycycline	• Relatively broad-spectrum oral agent that includes anaerobic coverage • Active against many MRSA and some gram-negatives; uncertain against *Streptococcus* species
		• Trimethoprim/Sulfamethoxazole	• Active against many MRSA and some gram-negatives; uncertain activity against Streptococci
Moderate [may be treated with oral or initial parenteral agent(s)] or severe [usually treated with parenteral agent(s)]	MSSA; *Streptococcus* species; Enterobacteriaceae; Obligate anaerobes MRSA *Pseudomonas aeruginosa*	• Levofloxacin	• Once-daily dosing; suboptimal against *S. aureus*
		• Ceftriaxone	• Second-generation cephalosporin with anaerobic coverage
		• Moxifloxacin	• Once-daily dosing, third-generation cephalosporin • Once-daily oral dosing. Relatively, broad-spectrum, including most obligate anaerobic organisms

Continued

Continued

Infection severity	Probable pathogen(s)	Antibiotic agent	Comments
		• Ertapenem	• Active against MRSA. Spectrum may be excessively broad
		• Levofloxacin or ciprofloxacin with clindamycin	• Limited evidence supporting clindamycin for severe *S. aureus* infections; PO and IV formulations for both drugs
		• Impenem-cilastatin	• Very broad-spectrum (but not against MRSA); use only when this is required. Consider when ESBL-producing pathogens suspected
		• Linezolid	• Vancomycin MICs for MRSA are gradually increasing
		• Vancomycin	• TID/QID dosing. Useful for broad-spectrum coverage. *P. aeruginosa* is an uncommon pathogen in diabetic foot infections except in special circumstances
		• Piperacillin-tazobactam	

(IV: intravenous; MIC: minimum inhibitory concentration; PO: per oral)

TABLE 11: Duration of treatment is based on location, severity, extent of wound with or without bone involvement.

Site of infection	Route of administration	Setting	Duration of therapy
Soft tissue only			
Mild	Oral	OPD	1–2 weeks, may extend to 4–6 weeks if has underlying osteomyelitis
Moderate	Oral or initial parenteral	Outpatient/Inpatient	1–3 weeks
Severe	Initial parenteral, shall switch over to oral on discharge	Inpatient	2 weeks, extends to 4–6 weeks if has underlying osteomyelitis
Bone involvement			
No surgery or residual dead bone postoperatively	Parenteral, switch over to oral		≥3 months

Offloading

Offloading is very important in management of DFUs. There are different offloading options available (**Box 1** and **Figs. 11A** to **D**). Completely or partially relieving pressure from the weight-bearing area of the foot by providing mechanical support aids in healing. Repetitive trauma and high plantar pressure on the ulcer bed are two primary reasons for the persistence of ulcers.

> **BOX 1: Various offloading options.**
>
> **Crutch/walking frame walking**
>
> **Non-removable:**
> - Total contact cast/instant total contact cast (**Fig. 11A**)
> - Bohler iron cast (**Fig. 11B**)
>
> **Footwear modifications:**
> - Half shoes
> - Clogs (**Fig. 11C**)
> - Insole "reliefs" (**Fig. 11D**)

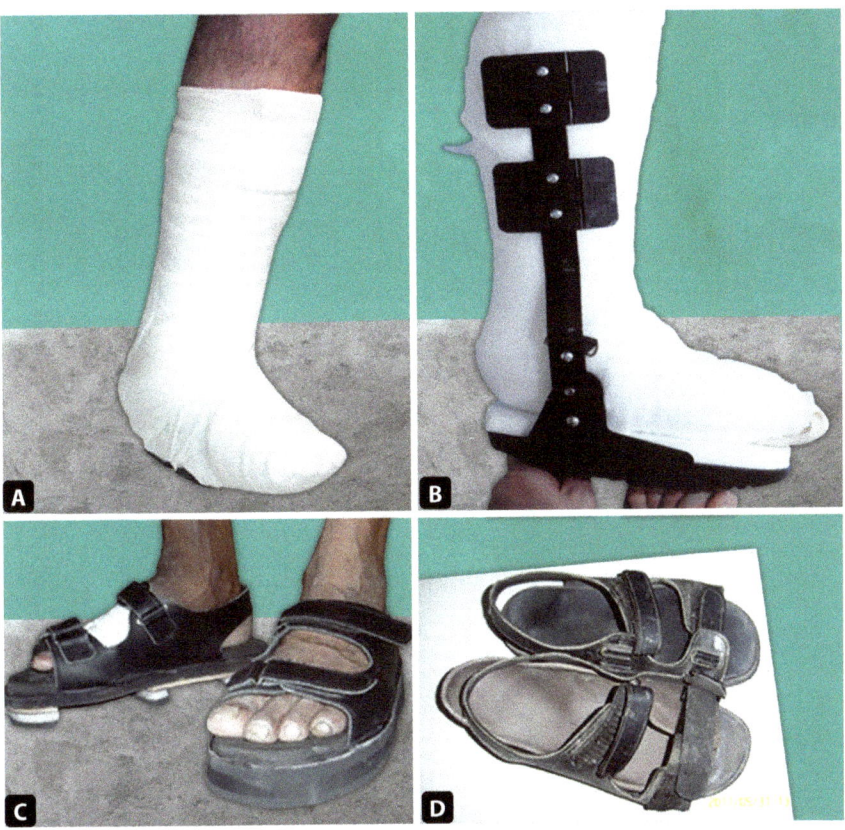

FIGS. 11A TO D: Different offloading options. (A) Total contact cast, (B) Bohler iron cast, (C) clogs, and (D) molded insole.

Diabetic Foot Ulcers: Clinical Approach

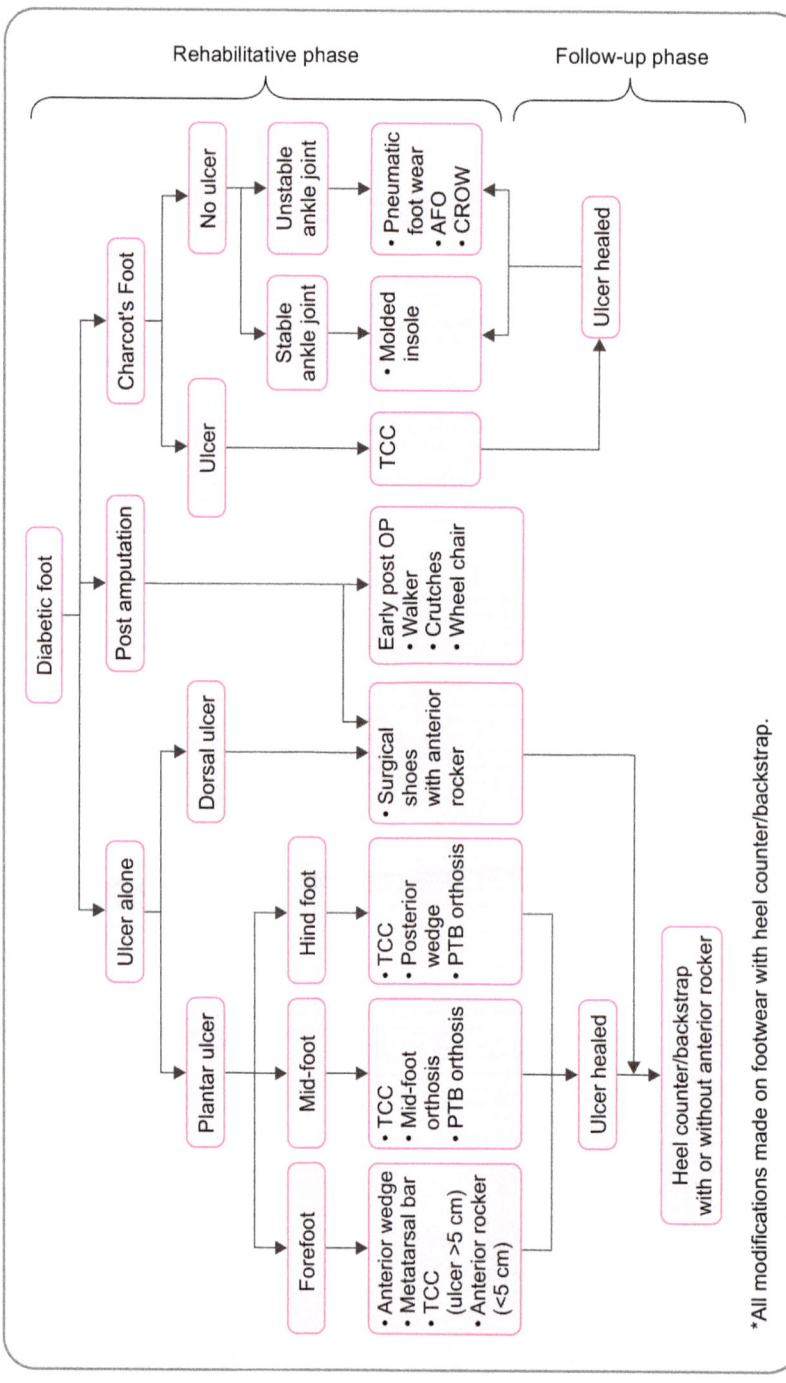

*All modifications made on footwear with heel counter/backstrap.

(AFO: ankle foot orthosis; CROW: Charcot restraint orthotic walker; PTB: patellar tendon bearing; TCC: total contact cast)

CASE SCENARIO

Our patient was advised to use walker and do daily dressing with saline. Once the ulcer started healing, she was advised to use customized anterior rocker for the amputated foot and microcellular rubber (MCR) footwear for the contralateral foot. She was educated on foot care and also to check her foot as well as foot wear daily to prevent future ulcers.

Health Education

Education regarding proper footwear and foot care is an important factor in wound healing. Patients should be emphasized on footwear, regular dressings, offloading, and frequent examination to look for signs of inflammation.

All the patients should be educated on four danger signs: Swelling, pain, color change, and breaks in the skin. Also, awareness to prevent recurrence of foot ulcers should be informed to all the patients.

CONCLUSION

Treatment of diabetes-related foot diseases needs a multidisciplinary team that includes a physician, surgeon, physical medicine and rehabilitation physician, specialist in orthotics and prosthesis as well as physiotherapist. Considering the paucity of these specialists in a single center, nonavailability of podiatrist in Indian setup, and the number of patients with diabetes and foot diseases, a primary care physician should be able to detect, treat, and offload the diabetic foot with the available resources, thereby preventing a future amputation. Only those who require specialized care should be referred to a higher center for further care and treatment.

REFERENCES

1. Singh N, Armstrong DG, Lipsky BA. Preventing foot ulcers in patients with diabetes. JAMA. 2005;293(2):217-28.
2. Boulton AJM, Vileikyte L, Ragnarson-Tennvall G, Apelqvist J. The global burden of diabetic foot disease. Lancet. 2005;366(9498):1719-24.
3. Viswanathan V, Thomas N, Tandon N, Asirvatham A, Rajasekar S, Ramachandran A, et al. Profile of diabetic foot complications and its associated complications--a multicentric study from India. J Assoc Physicians India. 2005;53:933-6.
4. Brod M. Quality of life issues in patients with diabetes and lower extremity ulcers: patients and care givers. Qual Life Res. 1998;7(4):365-72.
5. Most RS, Sinnock P. The epidemiology of lower extremity amputations in diabetic individuals. Diabetes Care. 1983;6(1):87-91.
6. Rathnayake A, Saboo A, Malabu UH, Falhammar H. Lower extremity amputations and long-term outcomes in diabetic foot ulcers: A systematic review. World J Diabetes. 2020;11(9):391-9.
7. Ebskov B, Josephsen P. Incidence of reamputation and death after gangrene of the lower extremity. Prosthet Orthot Int. 1980;4(2):77-80.

8. Armstrong DG, Lavery LA, American Diabetes Association, editors. Clinical care of the diabetic foot. 3rd edition. Alexandria, Virginia: American Diabetes Association; 2016.
9. Lipsky BA, Berendt AR, Deery HG, Embil JM, Joseph WS, Karchmer AW, et al. Diagnosis and treatment of diabetic foot infections. Plast Reconstr Surg. 2006;117(7 Suppl):212S-38S.
10. American Diabetes Association. Consensus Development Conference on Diabetic Foot Wound Care: 7-8 April 1999, Boston, Massachusetts. American Diabetes Association. Diabetes Care. 1999;22(8):1354-60.
11. Alexiadou K, Doupis J. Management of diabetic foot ulcers. Diabetes Ther. 2012;3(1):4.
12. Schaper NC, Apelqvist J, Bakker K. The international consensus and practical guidelines on the management and prevention of the diabetic foot. Curr Diab Rep. 2003;3(6):475-9.

CHAPTER 5

JEAN-MARTIN CHARCOT

Charcot was born in Paris, France in 1825. Being artistically gifted, he possessed a special skill to use his abilities and visual memory to form associations between patterns of disease. He is considered the founder of modern neurology. Some of his accomplishments include describing the brain's vascular supply, distinguishing tremors found in Parkinson's disease with those of patients with multiple sclerosis, and differentiating hysteria from epilepsy. He provided a complete clinical description coupled with the pathological changes associated with a variety of neurological diseases, allowing for their precise classification. In 1883, Charcot and his colleague Fere described involvement of the foot in patients with *tabes dorsalis*, coining the term "pied tabetique" which has come to be known as Charcot's foot. Charcot's foot can occur as a result of various peripheral neuropathies, the most common of which is diabetic neuropathy.

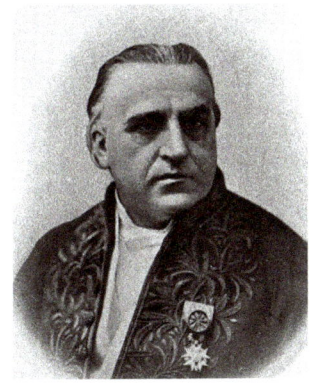

The Charcot Foot: Clinical Features and Management

Venkata Sandeep, Ilakkiya J, Bharathi K, Anand John Samuel G, Felix Jebasingh K, Nihal Thomas

CASE 1

A 49-year-old gentleman presented with sudden-onset, gradually progressive, severe pain in the left foot for 6 weeks with associated swelling. His pain was aggravated with movements and restricted his mobility. There were no systemic symptoms. However, he had symptoms consistent with neuropathy in the form of burning and numbness in both feet for over 3 years. He was known to have diabetes for 20 years and been on insulin for the past 10 years for his glycemic control. He had underwent laser therapy for advanced retinopathy. His neurological examination revealed distal symmetrical sensory and motor neuropathy. His left foot revealed swollen (prominent over the dorsum of the midfoot), warm, discolored foot with intact skin showing tenderness over the midfoot on palpation. He had no vascular compromise on clinical examination. His biochemistry revealed uncontrolled blood glucose with a high glycated hemoglobin (HbA1c) level. No features suggestive of infection were present (normal white blood cell count). His X-ray and the magnetic resonance imaging (MRI) of the foot are shown in **Figures 1** to **3A** and **B**.

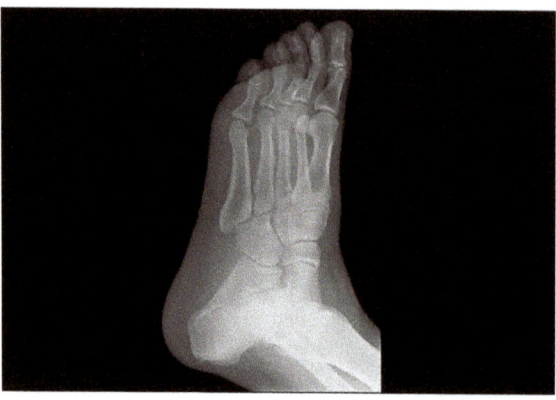

FIG. 1: Case 1: X-ray of the left foot with ankle joint, anterolateral oblique view.

The Charcot Foot: Clinical Features and Management

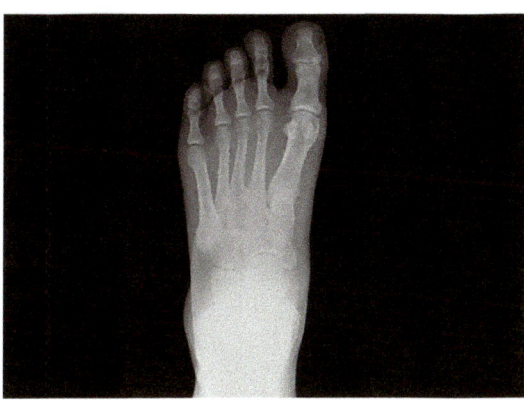

FIG. 2: Case 1: X-ray of the left foot, dorsoplantar view.

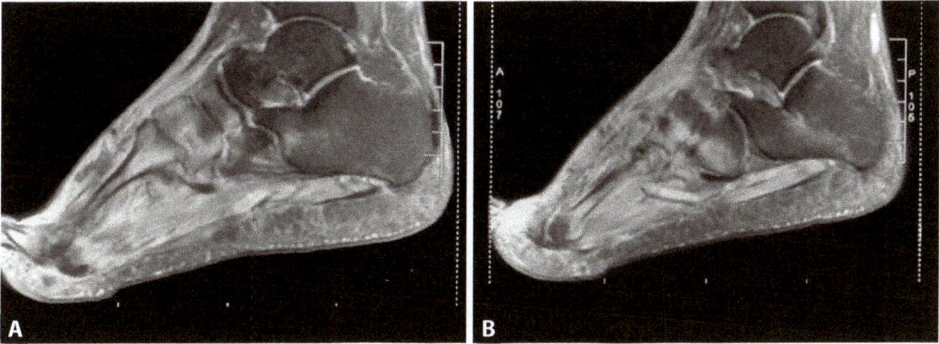

FIG. 3A AND B: Magnetic resonance imaging (MRI) of the left foot; (B) MRI of the left foot.

QUESTIONS

1. What are the differential diagnoses of this case?
2. What is the final diagnosis?
3. How do you manage this patient?
4. What is the role of pharmacological management in this case?
5. Is there a role for surgery in this patient?

CASE 2

A 54-year-old postmenopausal lady presented with complaints of swelling of the right foot for 9 months with associated pain over the last 3 months. There were no systemic symptoms. She had neuropathy in the form numbness in both feet for over 2–3 years. She had a history of ulcer requiring antibiotics in the past. She was known to have diabetes since 34 years of age, and on insulin for her glycemic control over

The Charcot Foot: Clinical Features and Management

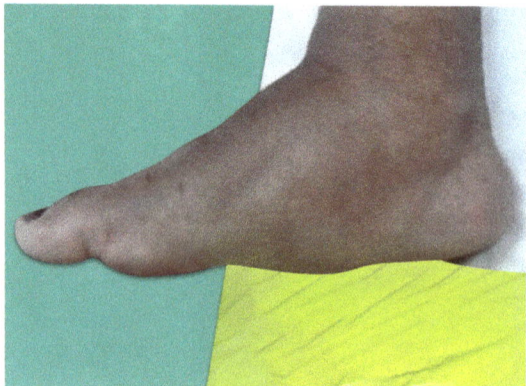

FIG. 4: Clinical image of the foot.

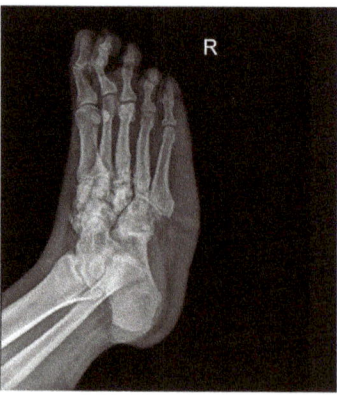

FIG. 5: X-ray of the right foot, anterolateral oblique view.

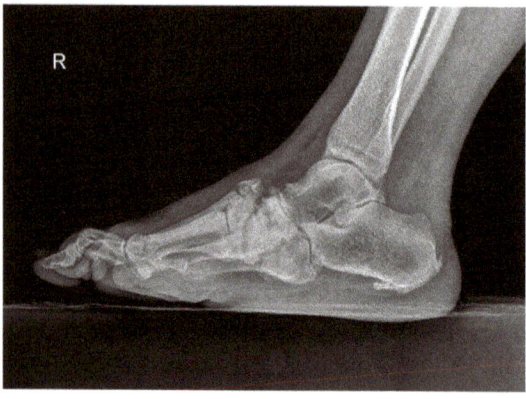

FIG. 6: X-ray of the right foot, standing lateral view.

the past 7 years. Fundus examination revealed moderate nonproliferative diabetic retinopathy in both eyes. Her neurological examination revealed bilateral distal symmetrical motor and sensory neuropathy with loss of protective sensation. Her right foot showed swelling over the plantar aspect of the midfoot with loss of the longitudinal arch (shown in **Fig. 4**). There were no other signs of inflammation. Her investigations were not supportive of infection (normal white blood cell count). The radiographs are shown in **Figures 5** and **6**.

QUESTIONS

1. What are the clues to diagnosis in this patient?
2. What is the final diagnosis?
3. How do you manage this problem?
4. What complications can be expected in this type of disorder, if left untreated?

INTRODUCTION

Charcot arthropathy (CA) is a non-infectious, progressive destruction of joints, most commonly involving the foot and ankle. It was first described by Jean Martin Charcot in 1868, in relation to tertiary syphilis (*tabes dorsalis*). Jordan was the first to note its relationship with diabetes mellitus (DM), in 1936. CA of the foot and ankle, a complication of DM, affects 0.1–2.5% of patients with DM. This prevalence increases to 35% in patients with long standing DM and apparent peripheral neuropathy.[1]

Frykberg et al.[2] estimated the involvement of various joints in CA which are as follows:
- Tarsometatarsal joint (40%)
- Naviculocuneiform, talonavicular, and calcaneocuboid-intertarsal joints (30%), and metatarsophalangeal and interphalangeal joints (15%)
- Ankle and subtalar joints (10%)
- Calcaneum (5%)

PATHOPHYSIOLOGY

There are several hypotheses that have been postulated on the pathogenesis of CA among patients with DM.
- The first one being the neurotraumatic hypothesis (the German theory), which is due to loss of proprioception following repetitive microtrauma.
- Second, the neurovascular hypothesis (the French theory), wherein autonomic neuropathy causes, denervation of arterioles, causing increased blood flow, thereby leading to osteoclast-mediated resorption and fragmentation. It also explains why patients with peripheral arterial disease are relatively protected from CA.
- Local inflammation causes series of changes which is elaborated below.

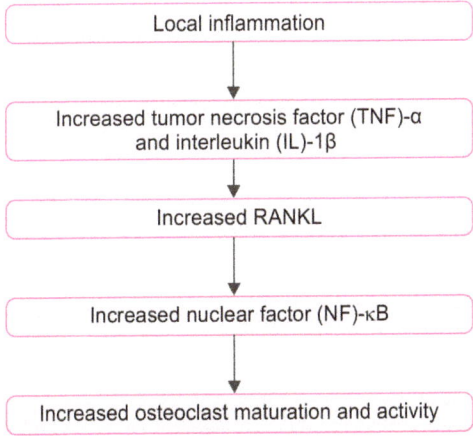

In normal joints, calcitonin gene-related peptide (CGRP), secreted by the healthy neurons, reduces the synthesis of RANKL and maintains joint integrity. Reduction

of CGRP due to neuropathy will indirectly increase the action of RANKL, thereby aggravating the disease process.
- Genetic factors such as polymorphisms of the gene encoding osteoprotegerin leading to predisposition for CA was also implicated.
- Other important factors include elevated plantar pressures and an increase in nonenzymatic collagen glycation.

From the literature, it appears that neurotraumatic theory applies more to type 2 diabetes mellitus (T2DM) than type 1 diabetes mellitus (T1DM). Conversely, the neurovascular theory appears to be more important for T1DM than T2DM.

CLINICAL FEATURES

The most common age group in which CA is found is in the fifth and sixth decades, affecting both genders equally, with a slight male preponderance. More often than not, no causative event can be identified.

Charcot's arthropathy is largely a clinical diagnosis. The presence of erythema, swelling, increased skin temperature, and joint effusion in an insensate joint is suggestive of Charcot's joints (**Fig. 7**).

The infrared cutaneous temperature monitor, used to detect foot skin temperature changes, is an accurate tool for the diagnosis of acute Charcot neuroarthropathy. It can be used in areas of the forefoot, midfoot, and hindfoot. A temperature difference of 2°C or more when compared to the contralateral normal foot indicates an active (acute) Charcot neuroarthropathy (**Fig. 8**).

A pilot study offered some hope regarding the potential value of corneal confocal microscopy as non-invasive biomarker for early stages of CA prior to the development of foot deformities by qualifying sub-basal nerve plexus changes.[3]

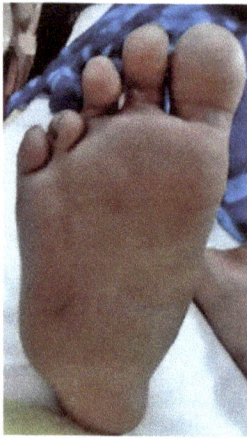

FIG. 7: Deformity in chronic Charcot foot.

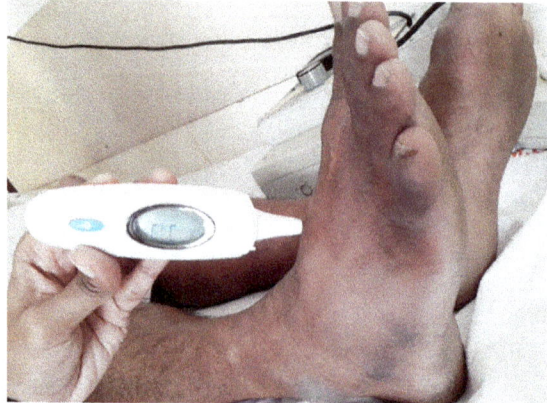

FIG. 8: Infrared thermometer for testing the temperature difference between the two feet. More than 2°C difference of that of the contralateral foot is significant.

CLASSIFICATIONS FOR CHARCOT ARTHROPATHY

Clinical classification—classified into the acute and chronic stage:
- *Acute (active) stage*: Erythema, swelling and redness of the foot usually affecting the midfoot. Pain may be absent or if it is present, it will be much less considering the degree of local inflammation. An infrared thermometer usually documents a 2–6°C temperature elevation of the affected foot when compared to the contralateral foot (**Fig. 8**). An MRI of the foot gives a definitive clue to clinch the diagnosis as the treatment of this condition needs a proper offloading to prevent further complications (**Fig. 9**).
- *The chronic (inactive) stage*: Signs of local inflammation subside progressively. The difference in skin temperature may not be appreciated. However, there may be obvious deformities (**Fig. 10**).

Eichenholtz Classification System modified by Shibata et al.[4]

Stage	Radiographic findings	Clinical findings
0 (prodromal)	Normal radiographs	Swelling, erythema, warmth
1 (development)	Osteopenia, fragmentation, joint subluxation, or dislocation	Swelling, erythema, warmth, and ligamentous laxity
2 (coalescence)	Absorption of debris, sclerosis, fusion of larger fragments	Continued but decreased warmth, edema and erythema, major bone deformity, and bone instability
3 (reconstruction)	Consolidation of deformity, joint arthrosis, fibrous ankyloses, rounding, and smoothing of bone fragments	Absence of warmth, absence of swelling, absence of erythema, and stable joint ± fixed deformity

Sanders and Frykberg classification (**Fig. 11**):
- *Zone 1*: Metatarsophalangeal and interphalangeal joints
- *Zone 2*: Tarsometatarsal joints
- *Zone 3*: Tarsal joints
- *Zone 4*: Ankle and subtalar joints
- *Zone 5*: Calcaneus

Brodsky's anatomic-based classification systems for CA,[5] modified by Trepman et al.[6] (**Figs. 12** and **13**).

Type	Location	Involved joints
1	Midfoot	Tarsometatarsal and naviculocuneiform
2	Hindfoot	Subtalar, talonavicular, and calcaneocuboid
3A	Ankle	Tibiotalar
3B	Calcaneus	Tuberosity fracture
4	Multiple regions	Sequential and concurrent
5	Forefoot	Metatarsophalangeal

The Charcot Foot: Clinical Features and Management

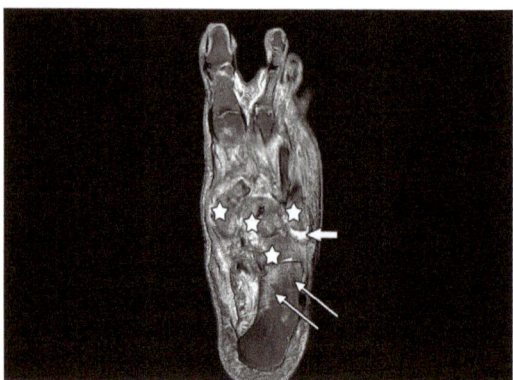

FIG. 9: Active Charcot foot: Zone 2 (tarsometatarsal) and Zone 3 (inter-tarsal) involvement showing diffuse bone marrow edema (shown with asterisk) of tarsal bones and base of metatarsals. Also, bone marrow edema is also seen in the periarticular region of the calcaneum (shown with the thin arrows). Joint effusion seen between tarsometatarsal joint (shown with a thick arrow).

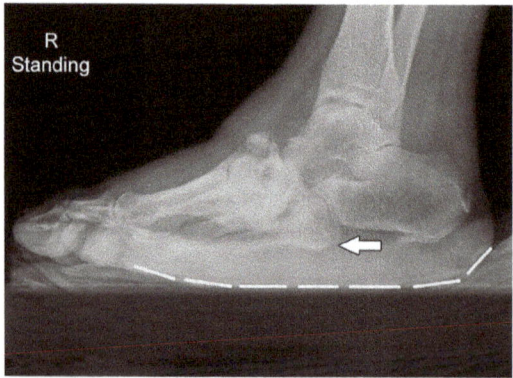

FIG. 10: Chronic Charcot foot with a rocker foot deformity. Cuboid forming the lowermost bone (shown with a thick white arrow).

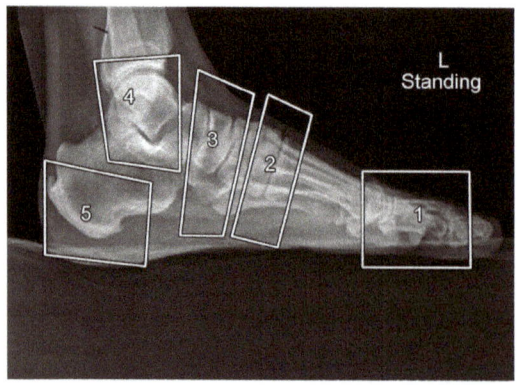

FIG. 11: Sanders and Frykberg classification: Representation of zones.

The Charcot Foot: Clinical Features and Management

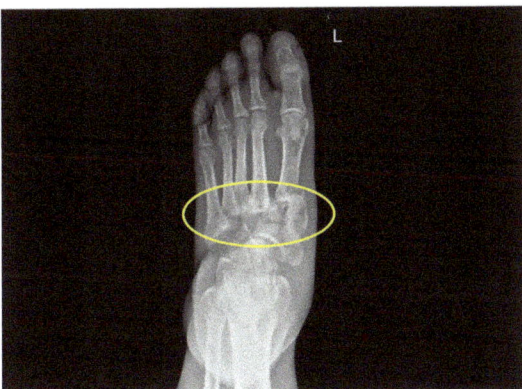

FIG. 12: Acute Charcot's foot: Zone 2—Joint space narrowing and destruction of metatarso-phalangeal joints.

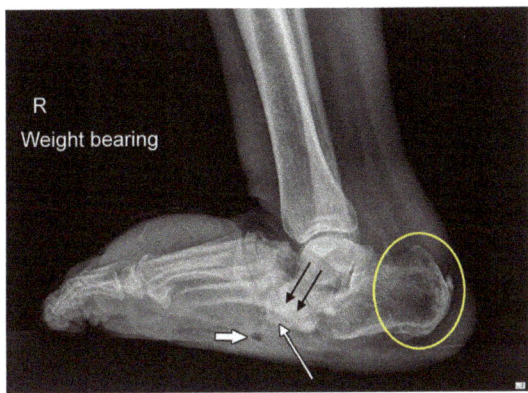

FIG. 13: Chronic Charcot foot with osteomyelitis, showing sinus tract (shown with a white thick arrow), sclerosis, and fragmentation of the cuboid (shown with thin white arrow), dislocation of the tarsal head downward (shown with the black arrows), osteolysis of calcaneus with posterior displacement (shown with a circle) indicating types 3, 4, and 5 Charcot foot. Soft-tissue swelling is also seen over the dorsum of the foot.

INVESTIGATIONS

Biochemical markers: C-reactive protein (CRP) and erythrocyte sedimentation rate (ESR) are usually normal in acute Charcot neuroarthropathy.

X-ray of the foot: Measurements[7] are used to assess the severity of the Charcot foot and are important during follow-up. It is important to take a proper view of the foot. One should advise an anterolateral oblique view as well as standing lateral view to measure the angles in the foot.
- *Meary's angle*: Angle between long axis of the talus and that of the first metatarsal; normal value is 0°. Meary's angle above 15° is taken abnormal (**Figs. 14, 15, and 20**).

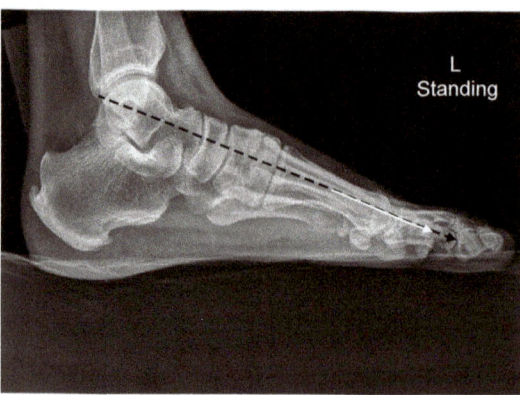

FIG. 14: Meary's angle: Angle between long axis of the talus (black dotted line) and that of the first metatarsal (white line). Above X-ray is that of a normal foot where the Meary's angle is 0°.

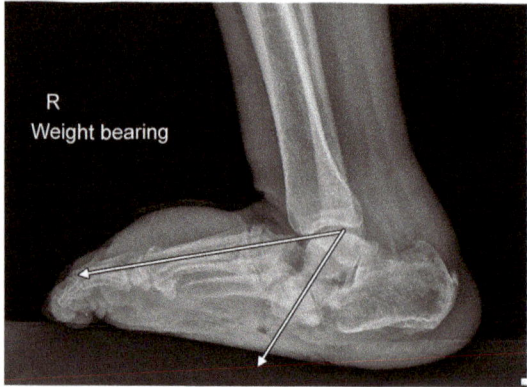

FIG. 15: Deformity in a chronic Charcot foot.

- *Calcaneal pitch*: Angle between a line extending from the plantar aspect of the calcaneus to the plantar surface of the fifth metatarsal head and the line extending from the plantar most portion of the calcaneal tuberosity to the plantar most portion of the anterior calcaneum. The normal value lies between 20 and 30°. A calcaneal pitch below 17° is taken as abnormal (**Figs. 16** and **17**).
- *Cuboid height*: Perpendicular distance from the plantar aspect of the cuboid to a line drawn from the plantar surface of the calcaneal tuberosity to the plantar aspect of the fifth metatarsal head. Normal value is 1.2 cm (**Figs. 18** and **19**).
- *Hindfoot-forefoot angle*: Best visualized in dorsoplantar (DP) radiographs. The hindfoot-forefoot angle is the angle between:
  ○ The longitudinal axis of the second metatarsal bone
  ○ *The bisection of another angle which is formed by the following two lines*: The long axis of talus and a line parallel to the lateral cortex of the calcaneus.
  The normal value is nearly 0°.

The Charcot Foot: Clinical Features and Management

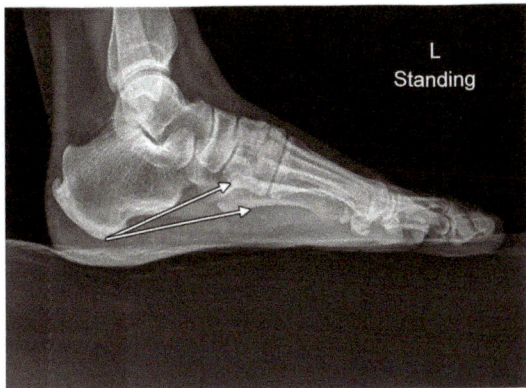

FIG. 16: Normal calcaneal pitch.

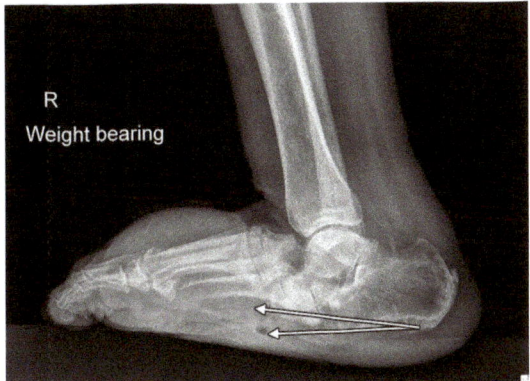

FIG. 17: Chronic Charcot foot with negative calcaneal pitch (abnormal).

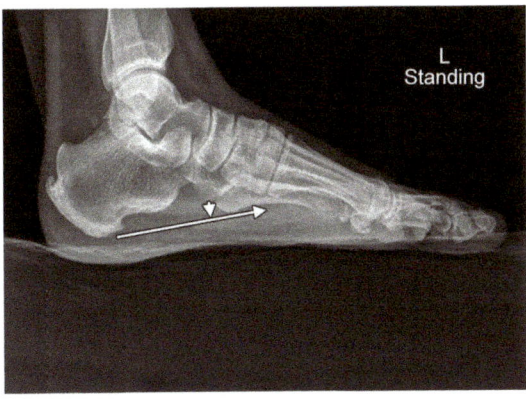

FIG. 18: Normal cuboid height.

The Charcot Foot: Clinical Features and Management

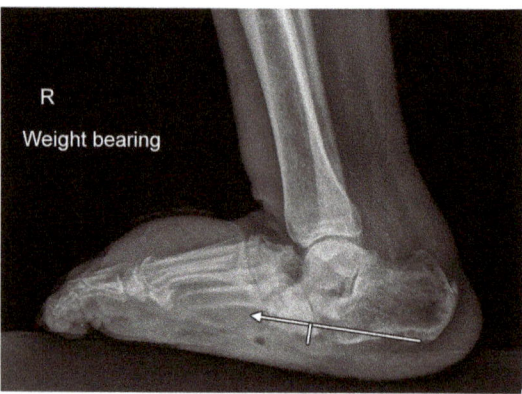

FIG. 19: Chronic Charcot foot with a negative cuboid height (abnormal).

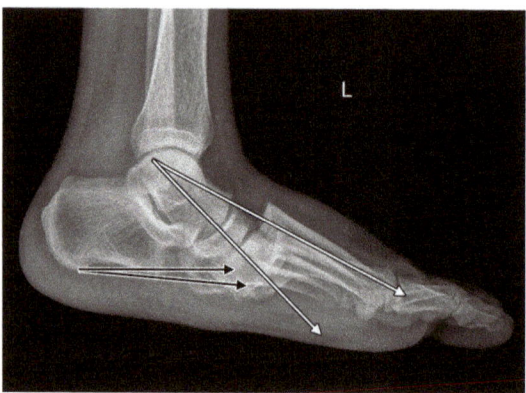

FIG. 20: Acute Charcot's foot: Zone 2 involved with collapse of the midfoot and dislocation of the metatarsophalangeal joints. Calcaneal pitch (Shown with the black arrows) decreased to 4° and the cuboidal height is negative with Meary's angle being 20° (Shown with the white arrows) confirming the diagnosis with a simple X-ray foot with proper views.

MAGNETIC RESONANCE IMAGING

Magnetic Resonance Imaging for Diagnosis of the Early-stage Charcot Foot

Magnetic resonance imaging is the best imaging modality to confirm the diagnosis during early stages of an active Charcot foot. Conventional radiographs can be normal during early stages of CA (Eichenholtz stage 0). Early signs of CA in MRI include bone marrow edema and soft tissue edema, joint effusion and microfractures (subchondral). No cortical fractures or gross deformity can be seen in early stages (**Figs. 9, 21,** and **22**).

The Charcot Foot: Clinical Features and Management

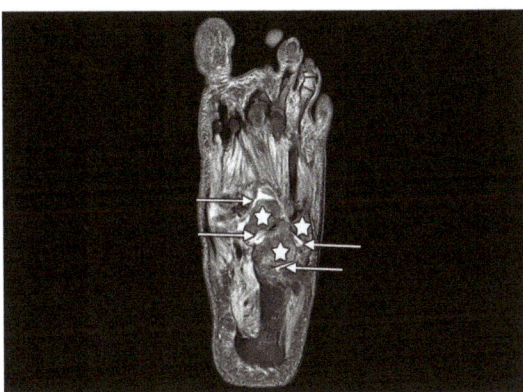

FIG. 21: Active Charcot foot-joint effusion (shown with the arrows) in metatarsophalangeal and intertarsal joints. Bone marrow edema is seen in the tarsal bones (shown with the asterisks) indicative of an acute Charcot foot.

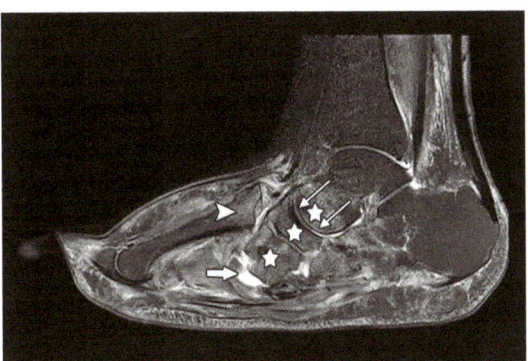

FIG. 22: Active Charcot foot: Bone marrow edema (shown with the asterisks) seen in talar head, navicular, cuneiform, base of metatarsal (shown with an arrowhead). Joint effusion (shown with a thick arrow) seen in the tarsometatarsal joint. Downward displacement of talar head (shown with the white thin arrows).

Magnetic Resonance Imaging of Middle- to Late-stage Charcot Foot (Fragmentation to Consolidation)

In an MRI of the foot, the joint destruction, cortical fractures, and joint dislocations are features that occur in the later stages of the disease. The presence of bone marrow edema indicates disease activity. Mid-foot involvement leads to superior and lateral dislocation of the metatarsal bones resulting in incomplete collapse of the longitudinal arch. The head of the talus is typically tilted inferiorly, the navicular bone usually dislocates into a medial and superior position, often with fractures and fragmentation. Prominent subchondral cysts are a typical feature of chronic Charcot foot. In addition, bony proliferation and sclerosis, debris, and intraarticular bodies can occur. In CA Fluid collections surrounding destroyed joints are usually huge (**Fig. 23**).

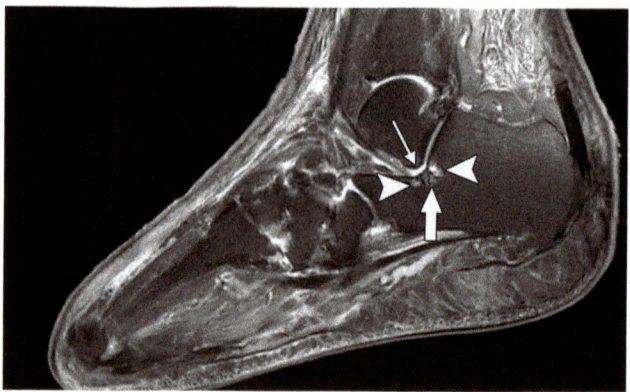

FIG. 23: Chronic Charcot foot: Zone 4 (subtalar joint)—subchondral cysts (shown with the white arrowheads), erosions, joint effusion (shown with a thin white arrow) and minimal bone marrow edema (shown with a thick white arrow).

Monitoring of Disease Activity with Magnetic Resonance Imaging

Magnetic resonance imaging of the foot is also the best imaging modality to monitor disease activity. Ideally, offloading therapy should be continued as long as a significant amount of bone marrow edema is seen on MRI. After a significant or complete disappearance of bone marrow edema, the total contact cast can be removed.

Chantelau and Grutznel Magnetic Resonance Imaging Classification for Charcot Foot

Stage	Grade	
	Low severity: Grade 0 (without cortical fracture)	**High severity: Grade 1** (with cortical fracture)
Active arthropathy (acute stage)	• Mild inflammation/soft tissue edema • No skeletal deformity • X-ray: Normal • MRI: Abnormal (bone marrow edema, microfractures, and bone bruise)	• Severe inflammation/soft tissue edema • Severe skeletal deformity • X-ray: Abnormal • MRI: Abnormal (bone marrow edema, macrofractures, and bone bruise)
Inactive arthropathy (becalmed stage)	• No inflammation • No skeletal deformity • X-ray: Normal • MRI: No significant bone marrow edema	• No inflammation • Severe skeletal deformity • X-ray: Abnormal (past macrofractures) • MRI: No significant bone marrow edema

Differences between Acute Charcot Foot and Osteomyelitis[8]

	Active Charcot foot	**Osteomyelitis**
Location of bone marrow abnormality	• Periarticular • Usually involves many joints and bones (tarsometatarsal joints and metatarsophalangeal joints)	• Usually involves a single bone with diffuse marrow involvement • Affects weight-bearing surfaces of the metatarsal heads, toes, calcaneus, malleolus, and cuboid (in rocker-bottom deformity) • Usually develops by continuous spread of infection from skin ulcerations and sinus tracts
Sinus tracts	• Usually not present	• Often present
Skin ulceration	• Can be present	• Often present • Often present in relationship to sinus tract
Fluid collections	• Present • Usually smaller than in case of infection, unless sinus tract is present	• Present • They are larger than in active Charcot's foot, unless a sinus tract exists over which the collection is drained (paradoxical decrease of size of the fluid collection) • Diffusion-weighted imaging (DWI) helps in differentiating abscesses from non-infected fluid collections
Subcutaneous fat	• Dorsal edema, plantar surface normal	• Often cannot be appreciated due to presence of cellulitis
Subchondral cysts	• Typical imaging feature in chronic Charcot's foot • The presence of subchondral cysts goes against the presence of infection	• Usually disappears in infection/osteomyelitis
Intraarticular bodies	• Intraarticular bodies usually seen in chronic Charcot's foot	• Often disappear during infection due to dissolution or obscureness by surrounding inflammation
"The ghost sign"	• Negative for ghost sign	• Positive: Outline of the bones "disappears" on T1-weighted images and "reappears" after contrast administration (or on T2-weighted images)

Computed tomography (CT) scan: During early-stage Charcot foot, CT does not play a role for imaging since bone marrow and soft tissue changes can be better visualized using MRI. However, CT may be used in later-stage Charcot foot for better visualization of bony proliferations and consolidation, or for planning of corrective surgery and treatment monitoring. Patients with renal compromise can preclude the use of intravenous (IV) contrast, limiting the use of contrast CT in this patient subgroup. CT and positron emission tomography (PET)-CT may be used as an alternative cross-section imaging tool in patients with contraindications for MR examination (pacemaker, severe claustrophobia, etc.).

COMPUTED TOMOGRAPHY SCAN

Advantages
- Used as an alternative cross-section imaging tool in patients with contraindications for MRI (pacemaker, severe claustrophobia, etc.).
- CT may be used in later stages of the disease for better visualization of bony proliferations and consolidation, or for surgery planning and treatment monitoring.

Disadvantages
- Less useful in early stages
- Use of contrast CT is limited in patients with renal dysfunction.

NUCLEAR MEDICINE IMAGING

Advantages
- It can be used as an alternative imaging tool in patients with contraindications for MRI (pacemaker, severe claustrophobia, etc.).
- Fluorodeoxyglucose-positron emission tomography (FDG-PET) is more useful than MRI in differentiating from osteomyelitis in view of higher specificity.
- PET-CT allows for the quantification of the inflammatory process in all stages of Charcot foot and can be used for follow-up and evaluation of treatment duration in addition to MRI.

The main disadvantage is that this is not available in all centers and is more expensive.

Bone scan (**Fig. 24**): Technetium-99m methylene diphosphonate (Tc-MDP) bone scan is useful for detecting and localizing abnormal bone, with high accuracy levels. Triple-phase bone scintigraphy has a high sensitivity but lower specificity for detecting active bony pathology. It cannot differentiate Charcot foot with osteomyelitis. There

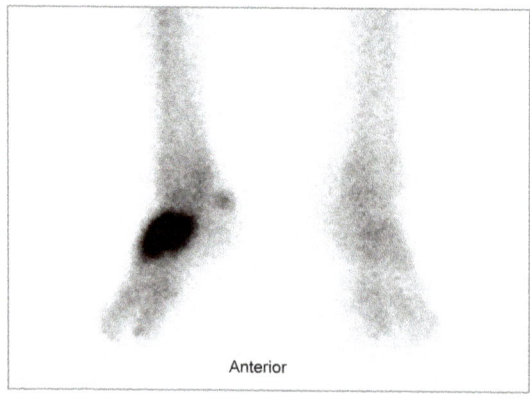

FIG. 24: Bone scan—right midfoot acute Charcot foot.

is an increased uptake in all three (angiographic, blood pool, delayed) phases. False-positive results are seen in fractures, tumors, and severe degenerative changes. It is false negative in those with vascular insufficiency.

Indium-111-labeled leukocyte scanning has the highest sensitivity and specificity for osteomyelitis. It can be used in cases of diagnostic dilemma.

BIOPSY

Bone biopsy is a potential tool for definitive discrimination between osteomyelitis and acute Charcot foot. The disadvantages are infection, excessive bleeding, fracture, or new onset of an acute Charcot process. So, generally it is a procedure that is discouraged.

MANAGEMENT OF THE CHARCOT FOOT

Eichenholtz stage 0: Frequent follow-up (serial radiographs) and diabetic education on foot care.

Eichenholtz stage 1 CN (development): Total contact cast—frequent follow-up with serial radiographs and casting until signs of inflammation have resolved.

Stage 2 (coalescence): Total contact cast or a molded total-contact polypropylene ankle-foot orthosis.

Stage 3 (reconstruction): (1) If the foot is plantigrade—custom inlay shoes; (2) If the patient is non-plantigrade or if there is a recurrent history of ulcerations—debridement, exostectomy, and correction (tendon lengthening procedures—generally of the Achilles tendon), fusion with internal fixation are the options.

Stage 3 with the presence of osteomyelitis—surgical debridement (with or without staged reconstruction with internal or external fixation) or amputation if there is a underlying life threatening sepsis .

Acute Charcot

Medical Management

Anti-resorptive drugs, such as oral bisphosphonates or IV pamidronate/zoledronic acid, have been used for the management of acute Charcot foot. However, no conclusive evidence exists to support their routine use. If given, a single dose of zoledronic acid or 70 mg of weekly alendronic acid for a period of three months is indicated.

Mechanical Offloading and the Role of Total Contact Casts

Total contact casting (TCC) is the preferred treatment modality for the management of acute CA as well as for those with chronic Charcot foot with an active non-healing ulcer.

The Charcot Foot: Clinical Features and Management

Casting decreases mechanical forces, edema and inflammation. It aids in the redistribution of plantar pressure, decreases bone and joint destruction and consolidates the progression of deformity. A close monitoring on a weekly basis with serial radiographs is essential until the active phase ends. Typically, changes in the Meary's angle would suggest fore- or mid-foot deformity development or progression and the need for more rigid means of holding the foot than casting.

Casting should be continued until resolution of swelling and redness or the temperature difference between the two feet is within 2°C and there is radiological evidence of good bony union. This period of casting could last from 4–6 months and is quite variable. Diabetic footwear should be prescribed with a custom-made orthosis to prevent recurrence after an acute episode has resolved.

The patient can later be changed to Charcot restraint orthotic walker (CROW) and after that to custom shoes or orthoses. A CROW is a total-contact ankle-foot orthosis, which is removable.[9]

In patients with chronic Charcot, one should prescribe the customized footwear depending upon the stability of the ankle joint. Patients with stable ankle joint (Stage 1–3) may be provided with a molded insole to prevent further worsening of the Charcot as well as future foot ulcers. In addition, if the ankle joints are unstable as seen in stages 4 and 5, the patient should be given ankle foot orthosis (**Figs. 25** and **26**) or pneumatic footwear/aircast boots (**Fig. 27**) to stabilize the ankle joint as well as in the prevention of future development of plantar ulcers.

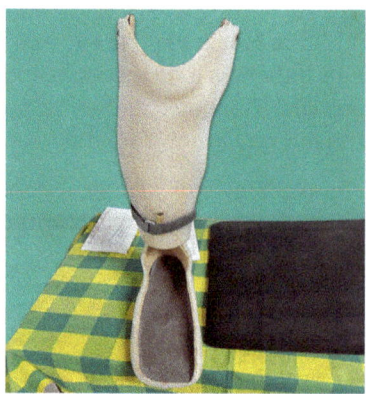

FIG. 25: Ankle foot orthosis.

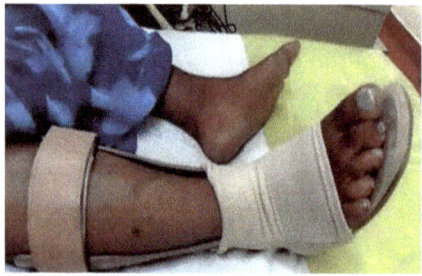

FIG. 26: Offloading of the Charcot foot.

The Charcot Foot: Clinical Features and Management

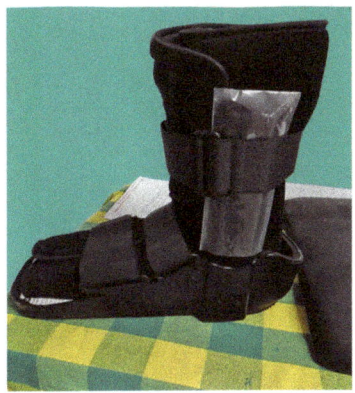

FIG. 27: Air cast boot/Charcot walker.

DISCUSSION OF CASE 1

Interpretation of an X-ray

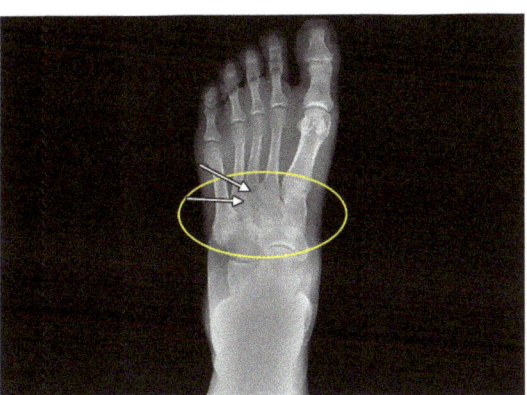

Interpretation of **Figure 2**: Acute Charcot—Involvement of zone 2 according to the Sanders and Frykberg classification (tarsometatarsal joints). Marked loss of the joint space and fractures (shown with the white arrows) of the base of third and fourth metatarsals.

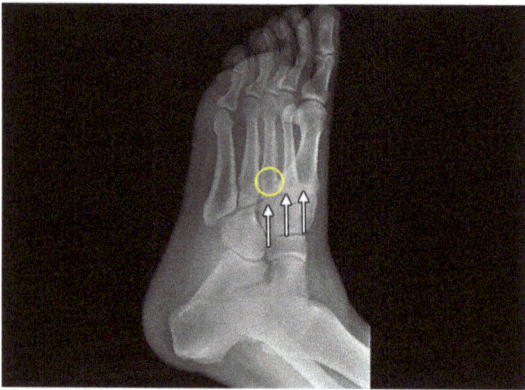

Interpretation of **Figure 1**: Acute Charcot foot—Involvement of zone 2 according to the Sanders and Frykberg classification (tarsometatarsal joints). Marked decrease in the joint space (shown with the white arrows). Fracture of the third metatarsal is evident (shown with a circle)—indicating Eichenholtz stage 1 (development).

Interpretation of Magnetic Resonance Imaging Foot

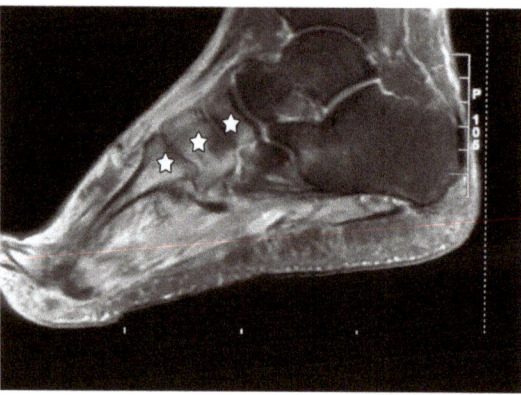

Interpretation of **Figure 3A**: MRI active Charcot foot—bone marrow edema (shown with the asterisks) seen in the tarsal (navicular and cuneiform) and metatarsal bones.

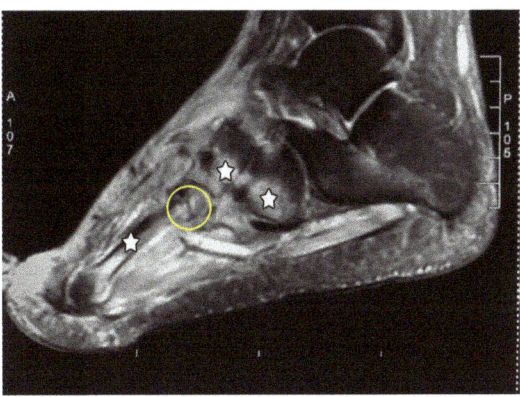

Interpretation of **Figure 3B**: MRI active Charcot foot—bone marrow edema (shown with the asterisks) seen in the tarsal (cuboid and cuneiform) and metatarsal bones. Base of metatarsal fracture (shown with a circle) representing grade 1 (according to Chantelau and Grutznel MRI classification).

What are the differential diagnoses in this case?

Cellulitis: Though it may be considered in the background of poorly controlled diabetes, the following features go against cellulitis—the absence of fever and other systemic symptoms. The white blood cell count is normal. Thus, cellulitis is unlikely.

Osteomyelitis: The skin is intact (no sinus tracts). No fever or other systemic symptoms. The white blood cell count is normal. The blood culture shows no growth. Thus, osteomyelitis is unlikely.

Gouty arthritis: though age, gender, and hyperuricemia are supportive, the following features go against gout: no involvement of the first metatarsophalangeal joint. Moreover, the duration of illness is 6 weeks (untreated acute gout usually resolves in 3-14 days). No systemic symptoms and signs of gout were noted. Typical radiological features of gout (erosions with overhanging edges, relative preservation of joint space) are absent. Thus, acute gouty arthritis is ruled out.

Acute mid-foot Charcot: Reasonably the most probable diagnosis in this case for the following reasons:
- Prolonged duration of DM (20 years)
- Poorly controlled DM
- Presence of B/L distal symmetrical polyneuropathy
- Absence of signs and symptoms suggestive of infection (i.e., absence of fever, normal white blood cell count)
- Involvement of the most common site [mid-foot: zone 2 involving the tarsometatarsal joints (Lisfranc joints)].

ANSWERS

What is the final diagnosis?
Mid-foot acute Charcot, Eichenholtz stage 1 (development)—fractures of base of third and fourth metatarsals, involving zone 2 (Sanders and Frykberg classification), MRI: active stage (bone marrow edema), and grade 1 (in view of cortical fractures).

How do you manage this patient?
Mechanical offloading using the total contact cast (TCC) is ideal. The alternatives include air cast boot (**Fig. 27**) or CROW (though these are usually considered after the subsidence of the active phase).

How would you follow-up the case?
Serial radiographs along with change of casting every 1-2 weeks. It usually continues for 6 weeks or should be continued until the clinical and radiological status improves.

What is the role of pharmacological management in this case?
Little evidence to suggest any available pharmacological therapies. However, bisphosphonates (oral as well as IV) may be tried.

What is the role of surgery in this case?
Surgery is generally avoided in the management of acute Charcot foot. However, it may be considered if the foot is refractory to offloading and immobilization (in the presence of deformities).

Is the treatment of acute neuropathic fractures different from non-neuropathic fractures?
The initial management of acute neuropathic fractures and dislocations is no different from other fractures.

DISCUSSION OF CASE 2

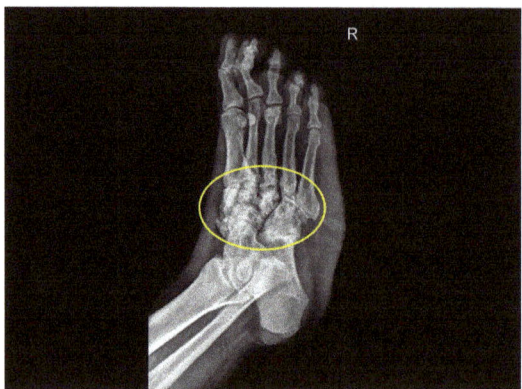

Interpretation of **Figure 5**: Chronic Charcot foot—According to Sanders–Frykberg classification, zone 2 (metatarsophalangeal joints) and zone 3 (intertarsal joints) are involved with decrease in joint space; osteolysis and fragmentation of the tarsal bones. Sclerosis (increased density) can be seen which is indicative of Eichenholtz stage 2 (convalescence).

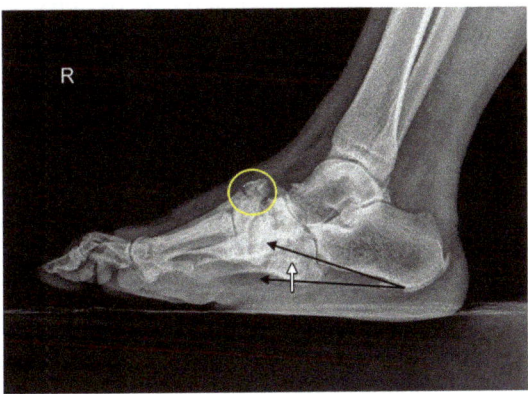

Interpretation of **Figure 6**: Chronic Charcot foot—According to Sanders–Frykberg classification, zone 2 (metatarsophalangeal joints) and zone 3 (intertarsal joints) are involved. Cuboid height is almost zero with cuboid occupying the lower most position (shown with an arrow). Calcaneal pitch is 13° (Shown with the black arrows). Sclerosis (increased density) and new bone formation (Shown with a circle) can be observed in tarsal bones indicating Eichenholtz stage 2 (coalescence).

ANSWERS

What are the clues to diagnosis in this case?
1. Prolonged duration of diabetes: 20 years
2. B/L distal symmetrical polyneuropathy with loss of protective sensation
3. Absence of signs of inflammation (chronic rather than acute)
4. The presence of a rocker bottom foot deformity
5. The pain is disproportionately low.

What is the final diagnosis in this case?
Chronic Charcot: Clinically, Eichenholtz stage 2 (stage of coalescence) involving zones 2 and 3 (Sanders and Frykberg classification).

How do you manage this case?
Patient has type 3, 4, and 5 Charcot foot, hence it would be advisable to use an AFO (to stabilize the ankle). If affordable, prescription of aircast boot or CROW device may be of added benefit.

What is the role of surgery in this case?
Since there is a rocker foot deformity (nonplantigrade foot), deformity correction may be tried. Various options include: (1) Exostectomy (excision of the bony prominence); and (2) Correction of deformity followed by arthrodesis (fusion of bones) with internal and external fixation. However, these surgeries require experience and good surgical skills and are less often successful on a long-term basis.

What complications can be expected in this case if left untreated?
This patient may present with recurrent non-healing plantar ulcerations in view of a rocker foot deformity which may lead on to osteomyelitis due to exposure of the bony prominences. All these may predispose the patient for an amputation.

REFERENCES

1. Schoots IG, Slim FJ, Busch-Westbroek TE, Maas M. Neuro-osteoarthropathy of the foot-radiologist: friend or foe? Semin Musculoskelet Radiol. 2010;14(3):365-76.
2. Frykberg RG, Sage RA, Wukich DK, Pinzur MS, Schuberth JM. Charcot arthropathy. Foot Ankle Spec. 2012;5(4):262-71.
3. Herlyn A, Prakasam RK, Peschel S, Allgeier S, Köhler B, Winter K, et al. Corneal subbasal nerve plexus changes in severe diabetic Charcot foot deformity: A pilot study in search for a DNOAP. Biomarker J Diabetes Res. 2018;2018:5910639.
4. Shibata T, Tada K, Hashizume C. The results of arthrodesis of the ankle for leprotic neuroarthropathy. J Bone Joint Surg Am. 1990;72(5):749-56.
5. Brodsky JW. The diabetic foot. In: Coughlin MJ, Mann RA, Saltzman CL, editors. Surgery of the Foot and Ankle. 8. St Louis, MO, USA: Mosby; 2006. pp. 1281-368.
6. Trepman E, Nihal A, Pinzur MS. Current topics review: Charcot neuroarthropathy of the foot and ankle. Foot Ankle Int. 2005;26(1):46-63.
7. Hastings MK, Johnson JE, Strube MJ, Hildebolt CF, Bohnert KL, Prior FW, et al. Progression of foot deformity in Charcot neuropathic osteoarthropathy. J Bone Joint Surg Am. 2013;95(12):1206-13.
8. Rosskopf AB, Loupatatzis C, Pfirrmann CWA, Böni T, Berli MC. The Charcot foot: a pictorial review. Insights Imaging. 2019;10:77.
9. Pinzur MS, Lio T, Posner M. Treatment of Eichenholtz stage I Charcot foot arthropathy with a weightbearing total contact cast. Foot Ankle Int. 2006;27:324-9.

CHAPTER 6

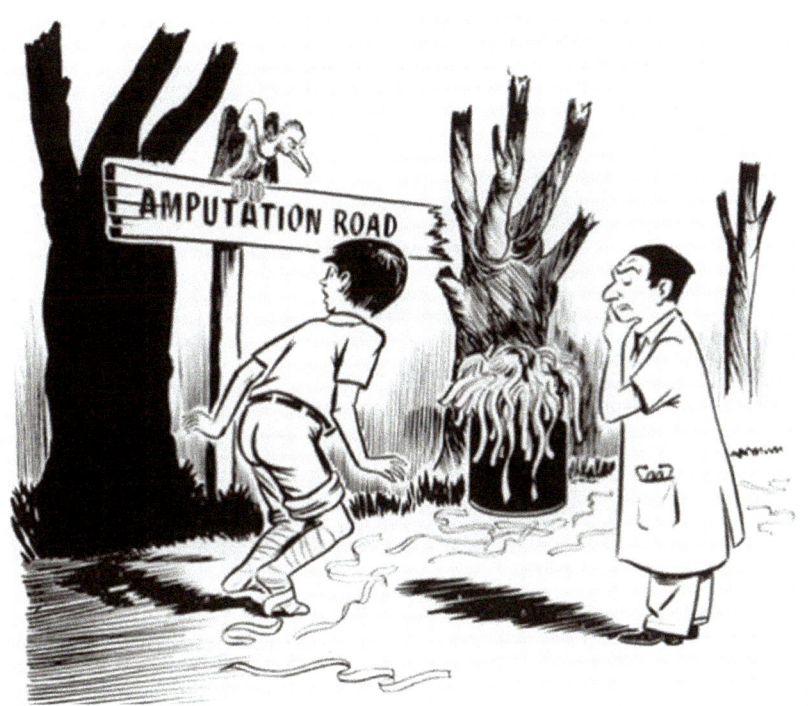

The cartoon depicts Paul Brand's 1966 warning that bandaging did not cure neuropathic ulcers in leprosy. It was later described that X-rays showing disintegration of the bones in a diabetic neuropathic foot were similar in appearance to those seen in leprosy.

Osteomyelitis of the Diabetic Foot

*Kelita George, Johns T Johnson, Kripa Elizabeth Cherian,
Shirly Jennifer N, Felix Jebasingh K, Nihal Thomas*

CASE CAPSULE

A 55-year-old lady having type 2 diabetes mellitus (T2DM) for over 12 years came with a history of an ulcer on the right great toe on the plantar aspect for the last 1½ months. It evolved following a thorn prick after barefoot walking. On examination, she had local gigantism of the left great toe along with an ulcer on the plantar surface (1 × 1 cm) with no features of active inflammation (**Fig. 1**). She had a callosity on the left second toe.

How will you proceed with the management?

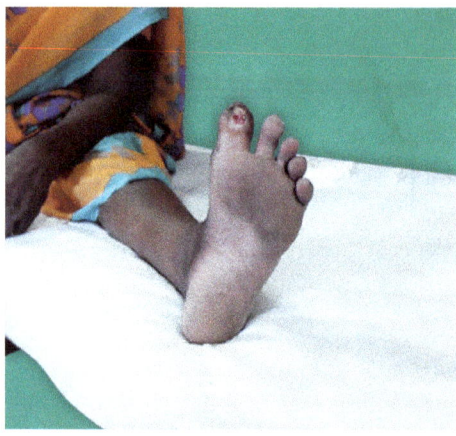

FIG. 1: Left foot showing local gigantism of the great toe with an 1 × 1 cm ulcer over the plantar aspect.

INTRODUCTION

Those with infected DFUs have an increased risk for multiple hospitalizations, amputations, and have higher mortality. Studies have shown that osteomyelitis is present in approximately 20% of patients with DFUs.[1]

Diabetic foot osteomyelitis (DFO) should be suspected in all patients with DFUs with clinical findings of infection, in chronic non-healing foot ulcers and in case of recurrent non-healing foot ulcers.[2] An early, accurate diagnosis is the cornerstone in the treatment of DFO, as well as in the prevention of minor and major amputations.

PATHOGENESIS OF DIABETIC FOOT OSTEOMYELITIS

Unlike other forms of osteomyelitis, in the diabetic foot hematogenous seeding is uncommon. Practically all the DFO results from contiguous spread of infection from the adjacent soft tissue. The initial soft-tissue infection is usually a complication of a neuropathic ulcer, or else from a surrounding ischemic soft-tissue loss or may be an ascending infection due to a penetrating injury. Osteomyelitis in DFO can affect any bone in the foot. Forefoot is the most common (90%) site for DFO, followed by midfoot (5%) and hindfoot (5%).

The pathogenesis of bone involvement commences as damage of the overlying periosteal tissue of bone by an overlying ulcer or through an ascending soft-tissue infection. This protective loss of the anatomical and physiological barrier allows microorganisms to gain access to the cortex of the bone. The infection further extends into the bone marrow through the Haversian system, leading to the involvement of medullary bone. This infection tracking beneath the periosteum causes necrosis of the underlying bone (sequestrum) and an overlying periosteal reaction with new bone formation (involucrum).

MICROBIOLOGY OF OSTEOMYELITIS

The epidemiology of microorganisms in DFU/DFO depends on the extension and the depth of wounds and the micro-environment of the ulcer. In view of contiguous spread, the causative microorganisms in DFO are similar to those isolated from soft-tissue infections. Infections are more often polymicrobial and rarely monomicrobial. *Staphylococcus aureus* (isolated in up to 50%), *Staphylococcus epidermidis* (25%), streptococci (30%), and Enterobacteriaceae (40%) are the most commonly detected bacteria. Among gram-negative bacteria, *Escherichia coli*, followed by *Klebsiella* and *Proteus*, are most common with *Pseudomonas aeruginosa* being isolated in rare circumstances. The swab from the DFO/DFU may rarely grow anaerobes. Most bacteria are multidrug-resistant or extended-spectrum β-lactamase-producing (ESBL).[3]

CLINICAL FEATURES

As in the aforementioned patient, the clinical features are rather nonspecific, since DFO can present with or without local signs of inflammation. In particular, patients with chronic osteomyelitis are largely asymptomatic. Fever with local inflammatory signs may suggest underlying cellulitis. Certain ulcer characteristics may suggest the possibility of underlying osteomyelitis:

- Accompanied by an erythematous, swollen ("sausage") toe (**Fig. 1**)
- A non-healing ulcer even after at least 6 weeks of appropriate wound care and offloading
- Wide and deep ulcer (**Fig. 2**)
- Ulcer discharging blood or serous fluid with or without bone fragments or with sinus (**Fig. 3**)
- Ulcer located over a bony prominence, showing visible bone (**Figs. 4A** and **B**)

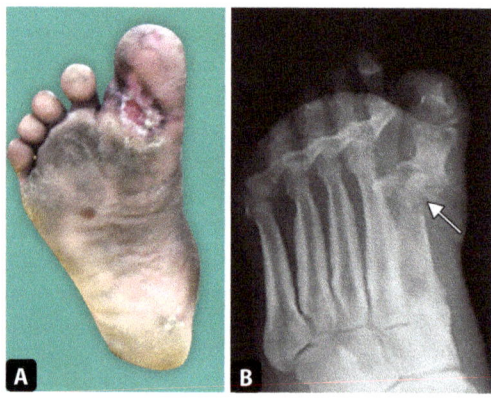

FIGS. 2A AND B: Deep ulcer with osteomyelitis confirmed with X-ray (shown with an arrow).

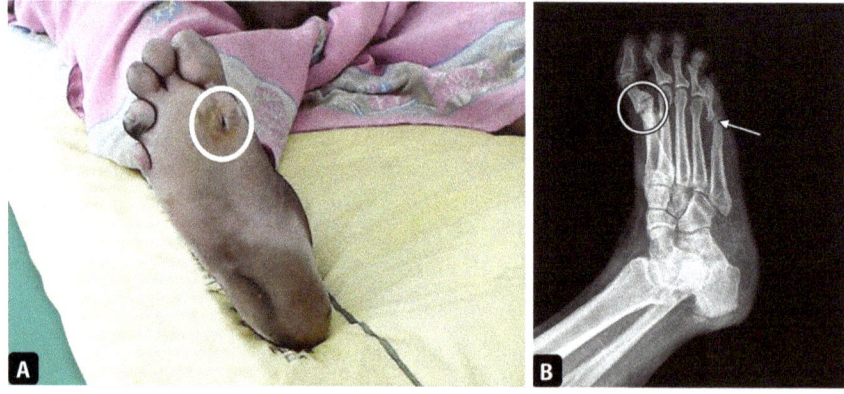

FIGS. 3A AND B: Sinus tract in the ball of left great toe with an X-ray of the foot with evidence of osteomyelitis in the first proximal metatarsophalangeal joint (shown with a circle) and a probable healed osteomyelitis of the fifth proximal metatarsophalangeal joint (shown with an arrow).

Osteomyelitis of the Diabetic Foot

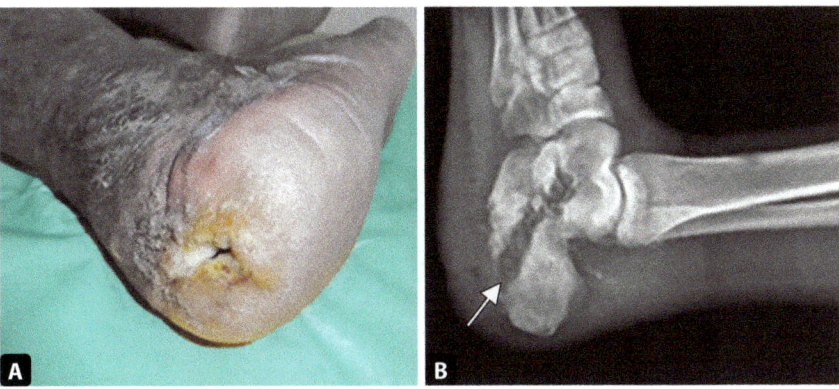

FIGS. 4A AND B: (A) Hindfoot ulcer and (B) infection tracking into the calcaneus causing osteomyelitis (shown with an arrow).

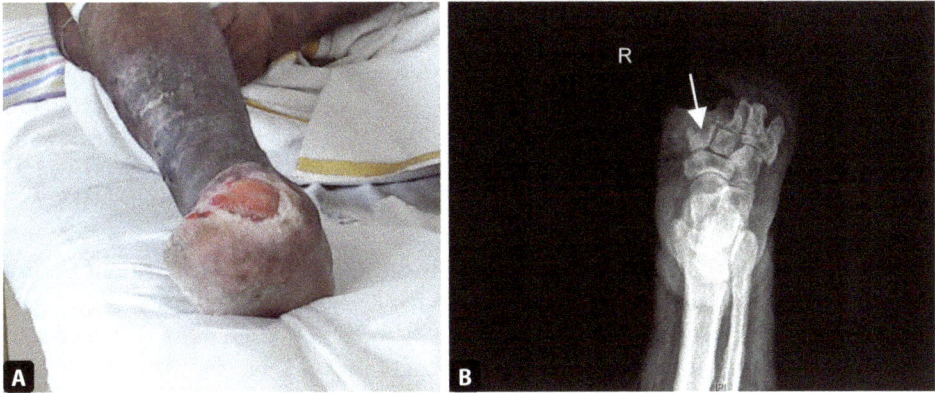

FIGS. 5A AND B: Patient with recurrent not healing stump ulcer (>2 cm²) with no obvious sinus and negative probe-to-bone (PTB), having osteomyelitis shown with an arrow.

Two clinical signs are predictive of osteomyelitis in the diabetic foot:
1. *Depth and width of the foot ulcer*: Deep ulcers (>3 mm) are more often associated with underlying osteomyelitis than superficial ulcers (<3 mm) (82 vs. 33%). Similarly, an ulcer larger than 2 cm² has a sensitivity of 56% and a specificity of 92% to be associated with underlying osteomyelitis (**Fig. 5**).[4]
2. *"Probe-to-bone test" (PTB test)*: PTB test is performed by probing the ulcer area with a sterile blunt probe. PTB is considered positive if the probe reaches the bone surface. PTB test has 87% sensitivity, 91% specificity, 57% positive predictive value, and 98% negative predictive value. Therefore, a positive PTB test is highly suggestive of osteomyelitis in the presence of infected ulcers. However, a negative PTB will not rule out an osteomyelitis (**Fig. 6**).[5]

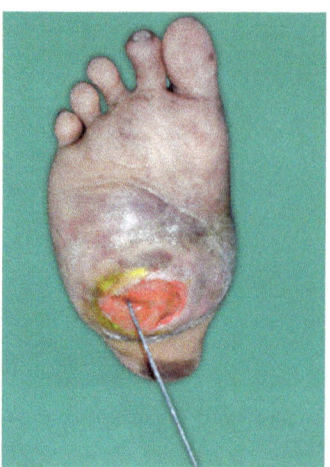

FIG. 6: Mid-foot ulcer with positive probe test.

LABORATORY INVESTIGATIONS

Serum inflammatory markers such as white blood cells (WBCs), erythrocyte sedimentation rate (ESR), C-reactive protein (CRP), and procalcitonin (PCT) are usually higher in DFO with active inflammation than with soft-tissue infections. However, WBC and procalcitonin may not be always elevated. ESR >60 mm/h and/or a CRP >3.2 mg/dL in the presence of an ulcer deeper than >3 mm are predictive of a DFO, although false elevations of CRP may be seen in those with underlying proteinuria and advanced microvascular disease. Therefore renal disease, which frequently occurs in these patients may also induce elevation of ESR and CRP. WBC count, procalcitonin, and CRP values generally return to their normal range in 3 weeks after treatment of both soft-tissue and bony infections, while ESR may remain persistently high in most patients with osteomyelitis (**Table 1**).[6]

IMAGING STUDIES

Radiological tests are usually required to detect bone involvement in case of suspected osteomyelitis without clinical signs of infection, to confirm the clinical suspicion and detect the affected bone/bones and to distinguish DFO from soft tissue infection.

X-ray

The plain X-ray of the foot is the first diagnostic tool used in screening, although clear signs related to osteomyelitis are generally not evident until 30–50% of the bone has been involved. This occurs after 2–3 weeks and thus it may be difficult to detect an osteomyelitic process during the initial phase with a plain radiograph (**Box 1**).[7]

TABLE 1: International Working Group on the Diabetic Foot (IWGDF) classification of infected diabetic foot ulcer.

Clinical classification of infection with definitions	IWGDF classification
Uninfected: • No systemic or local symptoms or signs of infection	1 (uninfected)
Infected: • At least two of these items are present: ○ Local swelling or induration ○ Erythema >0.5 cm* around the wound ○ Local tenderness or pain ○ Local increased warmth ○ Purulent discharge And no other cause(s) of an inflammatory response of the skin (e.g., trauma, gout, acute Charcot neuro-osteoarthropathy, fracture, thrombosis, or venous stasis)	
Infection with no systemic manifestations (see below) involving: • Only the skin or subcutaneous tissue (not any deeper tissues) • Any erythema present does not extend >2 cm** around the wound	2 (mild infection)
Infection with no systemic manifestations, and involving: • Erythema extending ≥2 cm* from the wound margin • Tissue deeper than skin and subcutaneous tissues (e.g., tendon, muscle, joint, and bone)	3 (moderate infection)
Any foot infection with associated systemic manifestations [of the systemic inflammatory response syndrome (SIRS)], as manifested by ≥2 of the following: • Temperature >38°C or <36°C • Heart rate >90 bpm • Respiratory rate >20 breaths/minute or $PaCO_2$ <32 mm Hg • White blood cell count >12,000/mm^3, or <4,000/mm^3, or >10% immature (band) forms	4 (severe infection)
Infection involving bone (osteomyelitis)	Add "(O)" after 3 or 4***

* Infection refers to any part of the foot, not just of a wound or an ulcer.
** In any direction, from the rim of the wound.
*** If osteomyelitis is demonstrated in the absence of ≥2 signs/symptoms of local or systemic inflammation, classify the foot as either grade 3(O) (if <2 SIRS criteria) or grade 4(O) if ≥2 SIRS criteria.

Source: Lipsky BA, Senneville E, Abbas ZG, Aragón-Sánchez J, Diggle M, Embil JM, et al. International Working Group on the Diabetic Foot (IWGDF). Guidelines on the diagnosis and treatment of foot infection in persons with diabetes (IWGDF 2019 update). Diabetes Metab Res Rev. 2020;36 Suppl 1:e3280.

Osteomyelitis of the Diabetic Foot

> **BOX 1: Features characteristic of diabetic foot osteomyelitis on plain X-ray.**
>
> - New or evolving radiographic features on serial radiographs, including:
>   - Loss of bone cortex, with bony erosion or demineralization
>   - Focal loss of the trabecular pattern or marrow radiolucency (demineralization)
>   - Periosteal reaction or elevation
>   - Bone sclerosis, with or without erosion (**Figs. 7** and **8A** to **D**)
> - Abnormal soft tissue density in the subcutaneous fat, or gas density, extending from skin toward underlying bone, suggesting a deep ulcer or sinus tract
> - Presence of sequestrum: Devitalized bone with radio-dense appearance separated from normal bone
> - Presence of involucrum: Layer of new bone growth outside previously existing bone resulting and originating from stripping off of the periosteum
> - Presence of cloacae: Opening in the involucrum or cortex through which sequestrum or granulation tissue may discharge
>
> *Source*: 2019 IWGDF Guidelines on the Prevention and Management of Diabetic Foot Disease.

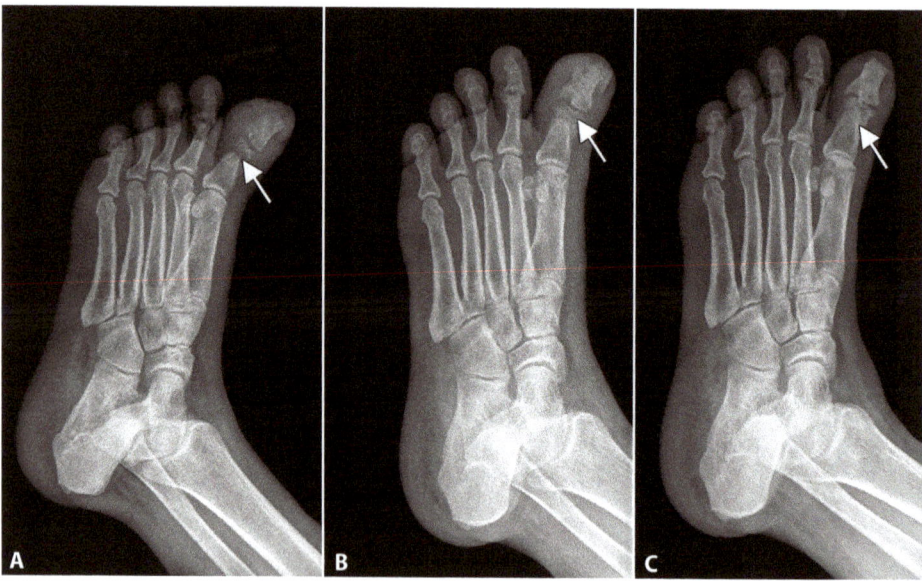

FIGS. 7A TO C: X-ray of the foot anteroposterior oblique view showing chronic osteomyelitis of distal phalynx of left great toe before and after treatment with antibiotics for a duration of 6 weeks.

MAGNETIC RESONANCE IMAGING

Magnetic resonance imaging (MRI) provides the greatest accuracy (combined sensitivity and specificity) for the detection of bone infection in the diabetic foot, among the currently available imaging modalities. The characteristic findings of DFO on MRI (**Figs. 8A to D**) are decreased signal intensity of affected bone on T1-weighted images and increased intensity on T2-weighted and post-contrast images. MRI also provides optimal definition of soft tissue infection, including detecting deep tissue necrosis, abscesses, sinus tracts, and higher inflammatory changes.[8]

It is not necessary to administer gadolinium to detect bony changes, but it increases the sensitivity of detection of soft tissue abnormalities.

The MRI of the foot has a high sensitivity (77–100%) and specificity (80–100%) in the diagnosis of osteomyelitis.[8]

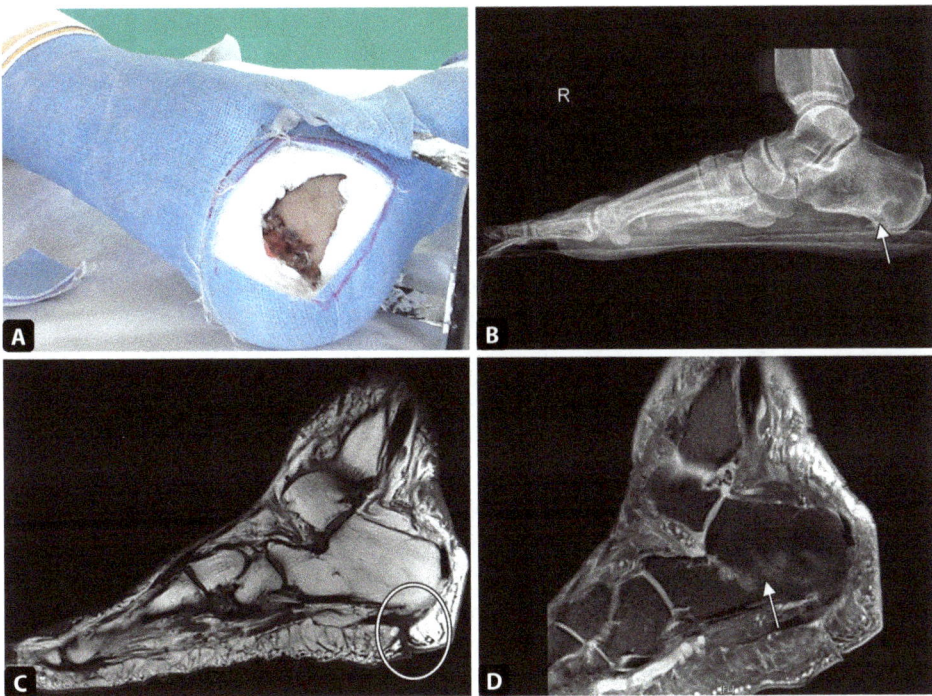

FIGS. 8A TO D: (A) Clinical image of the right Foot image showing an ulcer in the hind foot with a probe test being positive (Total Contact Cast-TCC in situ); (B) X-ray lateral view of the right foot showing a suspicious breach of the calcaneal periosteum (shown with an arrow); (C and D) T1-weighted image showing an ill-defined hyperintense sinus tract extending from the lateral aspect of the heel to the lateral calcaneal tubercle (shown with a circle) and marrow edema (shown with an arrow).

TABLE 2: Difference between the osteomyelitis and Charcot foot.

	Osteomyelitis	Charcot foot
Location	Mostly on the forefoot/heel (i.e., weight-bearing surfaces of the toes, metatarsal heads or calcaneus)	Mostly in midfoot
Site of bone/joint involved	Tends to affect a single bone with diffuse marrow involvement	Tends to affect several joints and bones with periarticular and subchondral involvement
	Soft tissue involvement—abscesses and sinus tracts may be present	Absence of soft tissue wound unless there is a superimposed osteomyelitis

Distinguishing the bony changes of osteomyelitis from diabetic neuro-osteoarthropathy (Charcot foot) may be challenging. It requires considering clinical information in conjunction with imaging. Clinical clues supporting neuro-osteoarthropathy, include a midfoot location and absence of a soft tissue wound, whereas presence of an overlying ulcer (especially of the forefoot or heel), either alone or superimposed on Charcot changes may suggest osteomyelitis. The presence of intra-articular bodies or subchondral cysts and involvement of multiple joints may favour neuro-osteoarthropathy; diffuse signal enhancement involving an entire bone, replacement of fat adjacent to abnormal bone, and presence of a sinus tract are features favouring osteomyelitis (**Table 2**).

Newer techniques such as magnetic resonance (MR) angiography and dynamic contrast-enhanced MRI may better distinguish Charcot foot from osteomyelitis.[9]

RADIONUCLIDE SCANNING

Scintigraphic examinations are generally more sensitive than plain radiographs, especially during the earliest stage of bone infection and follow-up. The low specificity in the discrimination between soft tissues and bone infection is a major limiting factor. Various radionuclide imaging modalities tried in DFO are:
- Bone scan using ^{99m}Technitium (^{99m}Tc)-MDP
- *Radiolabeled white cells*: Using ^{99m}Tc or ^{111}Indium
- ^{99m}Tc *WBC labeled-SPECT/CT*: Single-photon emission computed tomography and computed tomography
- Positron emission tomography-computed tomography (PET/CT) with fluorine-18-fluorodeoxyglucose (^{18}F-FDG) (**Table 3**)

BONE BIOPSY

Bone biopsy is the gold standard for the diagnosis of osteomyelitis, which provides histological and microbiological findings. The bone can be removed via a percutaneous approach, though not through infected skin or via open surgical procedures. Histological findings in osteomyelitis are bone erosion, marrow edema,

TABLE 3: Comparison between various modalities used in the diagnosis of DFO.

Imaging modality	Sensitivity (%)	Specificity (%)	Advantage	Limitation
X-ray	54	68	• Easily available • Low cost	Delayed diagnostic capacity
MRI	82.5	90	Good resolution	Reduced performance with severe ischemia
^{99m}Tc-MDP bone scan	80–90	30–45	High sensitivity	Low specificity
• ^{99m}Tc or ^{111}Indium • Labeled WBC	75–80	70–85	High sensitivity and moderate specificity	• Requires blood handling • Time consuming
^{99m}Tc WBC labelled-SPECT/CT	87.5	71.4	Good spatial resolution	Limited availability
^{18}F-FDG PET/CT	74	91	Good spatial resolution	High cost

(CT: computed tomography; SPECT: single-photon emission computed tomography; MDP: methylene diphosphonate; MRI: magnetic resonance imaging; PET: positron emission tomography; WBC: white blood cell)

Source: Pineda C, Espinosa R, Pena A. Radiographic imaging in osteomyelitis: the role of plain radiography, computed tomography, ultrasonography, magnetic resonance imaging, and scintigraphy. Semin Plast Surg. 2009;23(2):80-9.

fibrosis, necrosis, and presence of inflammatory cells (both acute and chronic). The bone biopsy also allows to identify bacteria involved in the infectious process and to evaluate the susceptibility to antibiotic therapy.

According to the Infectious Disease Society of America (IDSA) guidelines, obtaining bone tissue for culture and histology is likely to be justified when there is:
- Uncertainty regarding the diagnosis of osteomyelitis despite clinical and imaging evaluation
- An absence (or confusing mix) of culture data from soft-tissue specimens
- Failure of the patient to respond to empirical antibiotic therapy
- A desire to use antibiotic agents that may be especially effective for osteomyelitis but have a high potential for selecting resistant organisms (e.g., rifampin and fluoroquinolones).

TREATMENT

Surgical resection of infected bone has long been the standard treatment of osteomyelitis. Over the past two decades, evidence from several retrospective and prospective studies have demonstrated that in properly selected patients, antibiotic therapy alone is effective.[10] In the absence of soft tissue infectious complications such as extensive necrosis or gangrene, deep abscesses, tissue gas, or a compartment syndrome, most DFO do not require surgical intervention.

Osteomyelitis of the Diabetic Foot

> **BOX 2: Indications for nonsurgical treatment in diabetic foot osteomyelitis.**
> - No persisting sepsis (after 48–72 hours if on treatment)
> - Patient can receive and tolerate appropriate antibiotic therapy
> - The degree of bony destruction has not caused irreversible compromise to mechanics of the foot (bearing in mind potential for bony reconstitution)
> - Patient prefers to avoid surgery
> - Patient comorbidities confer high risk to surgery
> - No contraindications to prolonged antibiotic therapy (e.g., high risk for *C. difficile* infection)
> - Surgery not otherwise required to deal with adjacent soft tissue infection or necrosis
>
> *Source*: Lipsky BA, Berendt AR, Cornia PB, Pile JC, Peters EJG, Armstrong GD, et al. 2012 Infectious Diseases Society of America clinical practice guideline for the diagnosis and treatment of diabetic foot infections. Clin Infect Dis. 2012:54(12):e132-73.

> **BOX 3: Indications for bone resection in diabetic foot osteomyelitis.**
> - Persistent sepsis syndrome with no other explanation
> - Inability to deliver or patient to tolerate appropriate antibiotic therapy
> - Progressive bony deterioration despite appropriate therapy
> - Degree of bony destruction irretrievably compromises mechanics of foot
> - Patient prefers to avoid prolonged antibiotics or to hasten wound healing
> - To achieve a manageable soft tissue wound or primary closure
> - Prolonged antibiotics therapy is relatively contraindicated or is not likely to be effective (e.g., presence of renal failure)
>
> *Source*: Lipsky BA, Berendt AR, Cornia PB, Pile JC, Peters EJG, Armstrong GD, et al. 2012 Infectious Diseases Society of America clinical practice guideline for the diagnosis and treatment of diabetic foot infections. Clin Infect Dis. 2012:54(12):e132-73.

Performing any required surgery as an elective procedure allows the treating team to prepare and educate the patient well, decide which diagnostic studies are needed, and to select appropriate empirical antibiotic therapy (**Boxes 2** and **3**).

DURATION OF ANTIBIOTICS

The choice of antibiotics is given in detail in the Chapter 4: Diabetic Foot Ulcers: Clinical Approach.

There is no general consensus regarding the duration of antibiotics. The IWGDF guideline has suggested 6 weeks of antibiotic therapy if the infected bone was not removed by surgery and no more than a week if infected bone was resected (**Table 4**).

According to the IDSA guidelines, the duration of antibiotic therapy is as follows in **Table 4**.

TABLE 4: Duration of antibiotic therapy.

Bone or joint involvement	Duration of antibiotics
No residual infected tissue	2–5 days
Residual infected soft tissue (but no bone)	1–3 weeks
Residual infected but viable bone	4–6 weeks
No surgery or residual dead bone post operatively	≥3 months

CONCLUSION

- In a person with diabetes mellitus and foot infection, a detailed clinical examination including the probe-to-bone test can predict osteomyelitis.
- Combination of PTB test with X-ray improves the sensitivity and specificity in the diagnosis of DFO.
- If a plain X-ray and clinical and laboratory findings are compatible with osteomyelitis, no further imaging of the foot is required to establish the diagnosis.
- If the diagnosis of osteomyelitis remains in doubt, advanced imaging study such as magnetic resonance imaging (MRI) scan can be useful.
- Bone biopsy is the gold standard for the diagnosis of osteomyelitis, which provides histological and microbiological findings, but is rarely required.
- In a patient with uncomplicated osteomyelitis, treating with antibiotic therapy without surgical resection of bone will suffice.
- When there is a concomitant soft tissue infection, urgent surgery and if required amputation of the affected limb can be lifesaving.
- Treat DFO with antibiotic therapy for no longer than 6 weeks. If the infection does not clinically improve within the first 2-4 weeks, reconsider the need for selecting an alternative antibiotic regimen, collecting a bone specimen for culture or undertaking surgical resection.
- If debridement had been performed in DFO, there is no soft-tissue infection and all the infected bone has been surgically removed, antibiotic therapy should be given for just a few days.
- In case of associated cellulitis, those with DFO should be given parenteral therapy for 5-7 days, and then switch to an oral antibiotic regimen that has high bioavailability for a total duration of at least 6 weeks.

CASE DISCUSSION

At the beginning of the chapter, we began our discussion with a capsule of a patient. The X-ray of her foot showed evidence of osteomyelitis of the distal phalanx of the right great toe (**Fig. 7A**).

She was started on oral amoxicillin and clavulanic acid 625 mg, thrice daily, for 6 weeks. She was also advised to use footwear with an anterior rocker modification. During follow-up, after 6 weeks, it was seen that her ulcer had healed completely.

REFERENCES

1. Lavery LA, Armstrong DG, Wunderlich RP, Mohler MJ, Wendel CS, Lipsky BA. Risk factors for foot infections in individuals with diabetes. Diabetes Care. 2006;29(6):1288-93.
2. Berendt AR, Peters EJG, Bakker K, Embil JM, Eneroth M, Hinchliffe RJ, et al. Diabetic foot osteomyelitis: a progress report on diagnosis and a systematic review of treatment. Diabetes Metab Res Rev. 2008;24 Suppl 1:S145-61.
3. Eady EA, Cove JH. Staphylococcal resistance revisited: community-acquired methicillin resistant *Staphylococcus aureus*--an emerging problem for the management of skin and soft tissue infections. Curr Opin Infect Dis. 2003;16(2):103-24.
4. Lipsky BA, Aragón-Sánchez J, Diggle M, Embil J, Kono S, Lavery L, et al. IWGDF guidance on the diagnosis and management of foot infections in persons with diabetes. Diabetes Metab Res Rev. 2016;32 Suppl 1:45-74.
5. Morales Lozano R, González Fernández ML, Martinez Hernández D, Beneit Montesinos JV, Guisado Jiménez S, Gonzalez Jurado MA. Validating the probe-to-bone test and other tests for diagnosing chronic osteomyelitis in the diabetic foot. Diabetes Care. 2010;33(10):2140-5.
6. Michail M, Jude E, Liaskos C, Karamagiolis S, Makrilakis K, Dimitroulis D, et al. The performance of serum inflammatory markers for the diagnosis and follow-up of patients with osteomyelitis. Int J Low Extrem Wounds. 2013;12(2):94-9.
7. Hartemann-Heurtier A, Senneville E. Diabetic foot osteomyelitis. Diabetes Metab. 2008;34(2):87-95.
8. Ledermann HP, Schweitzer ME, Morrison WB. Nonenhancing tissue on MR imaging of pedal infection: characterization of necrotic tissue and associated limitations for diagnosis of osteomyelitis and abscess. AJR Am J Roentgenol. 2002;178(1):215-22.
9. Martín Noguerol T, Luna Alcalá A, Beltrán LS, Gómez Cabrera M, Broncano Cabrero J, Vilanova JC. Advanced MR imaging techniques for differentiation of neuropathic arthropathy and osteomyelitis in the diabetic foot. Radiogr Rev Publ Radiol Soc N Am Inc. 2017;37(4):1161-80.
10. Senneville E, Lombart A, Beltrand E, Valette M, Legout L, Cazaubiel M, et al. Outcome of diabetic foot osteomyelitis treated nonsurgically: a retrospective cohort study. Diabetes Care. 2008;31(4):637-42.

CHAPTER 7

WILLIAM PAVY

Frederick William Pavy was born on May 29, 1829 in Wiltshire, England. He received his MB degree from London University, with honors in physiology and medicine, and his MD degree in 1853. His later work was on central nervous system lesions, leading to diabetes. He is the author of the classical book, "Researches on the Nature and Treatment of Diabetes", which was published almost 100 years ago. The book contains his initial experimental work and his theories on diabetes. Pavy carefully described phenomena such as allodynia, nocturnal exacerbation of symptoms, and hyperalgesia, especially in the lower extremities and foot.

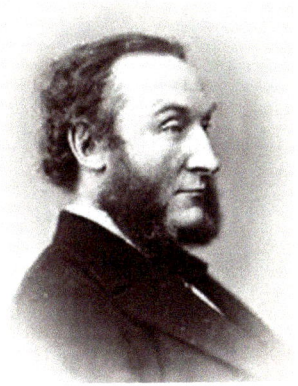

Peripheral Vascular Disease: Clinical Approach

Albert Abhinay Kota, Sunil Agarwal (Late)

INTRODUCTION

The global burden of diabetes has increased rapidly over the past decade. Diabetes and smoking are the strongest risk factors for peripheral arterial disease (PAD) with an odds ratio of 2.72 and 1.88, respectively. The incidence of PAD among patients with diabetes is increasing worldwide, and estimates between 10 and 40% are reported. Over 50% are asymptomatic or present with atypical symptoms as a result of decreased pain perception from peripheral neuropathy. The lifetime risk of developing a foot ulcer in people with diabetes is nearly 25%, and PAD is often related. PAD is seen in around 50% of those with a diabetic foot ulcer (DFU) and plays a role in 70% of the mortality among diabetic patients.[1]

Peripheral arterial disease independently increases the risk of non-healing ulcers, infection and leg amputation. In the EURODIALE study, patients with a foot ulcer and PAD had healing rates which were worse (69% vs. 84%) and higher major amputation rates (8% vs. 2%). In people with diabetes, PAD can remain undiagnosed until they present with severe tissue loss, progressing rapidly to limb loss. Claudication may be unusual in people with diabetes due to concomitant peripheral neuropathy, which diminishes sensory perception. Infrapopliteal occlusive disease with heavy calcification is the classic picture of diabetic arterial disease.

The most important risk factors associated with development of a new foot ulcer include a previous history of foot ulceration, reduced sensation, and the absence of any single pedal pulse. Amputation is largely a preventable complication of diabetes; over 85% of major amputations in people with diabetes are preceded by foot ulceration.

PATHOPHYSIOLOGY

It was previously thought that diabetes was an occlusive small arterial disease with lesions at the level of the arterioles. There is no evidence of diabetes specific arteriolar or capillary occlusive small vessel disease. Microcirculatory disturbances in diabetes are seen in neuropathy, retinopathy, and nephropathy, and are classically associated with endothelial dysfunction leading to thickening of the capillary basement membrane and reduction in capillary size. Large vessel disease is a consequence of atherosclerosis and vascular calcification. People with diabetes tend to have more diffuse atherosclerotic lesions that are multilevel, and particularly severe in tibial arteries with a high prevalence of long occlusions. There are often multiple crural vessel involvement which is combined with extensive medial arterial calcification. The formation of collateral vessels in response to large vessel occlusion is impaired in diabetes. Angiogenesis and other mechanisms to overcome ischemic response to the extremities are impaired. Despite the sparing of small pedal arteries in diabetes, there are unique changes in the microcirculation; the endothelium plays a central role and its malfunction is the hallmark of diabetic microvascular disease.

DIAGNOSIS

The diagnosis of PAD in people with a DFU is of critical importance. Assessing flow and perfusion can provide information on the hemodynamic consequences of arterial lesions and may help predict wound healing. Failure to diagnose and treat underlying PAD is a major cause of amputation in people with diabetes.

Investigations to Assess Foot Perfusion

Non-invasive Tests
- Ankle brachial pressure index (ABPI)
- Toe brachial index (TBI)
- Toe pressure (TP)
- Transcutaneous oxygen pressure (TcPO$_2$)
- Pulse wave recording waveforms (PVR)
- Photoplethysmogram (PPG)
- Skin perfusion pressure (SPP)
- Color Doppler ultrasound (CDUS)

Invasive Tests
Angiogram
- Digital subtraction angiogram (DSA)
- Computed tomography angiogram (CTA)
- Contrast-enhanced magnetic resonance angiogram (CE-MRA)

Non-invasive imaging modalities include ABPI, TBI, TP, and TcPO$_2$. The presence of heavy medial arterial calcification renders the lower leg and pedal arteries less compressible/compliant during cuff inflation, resulting in an inaccurate ABPI. Therefore, an individual with diabetes and a normal ABPI, may still have PAD. The sensitivity and specificity of ABPI as a screening tool in detecting PAD in people

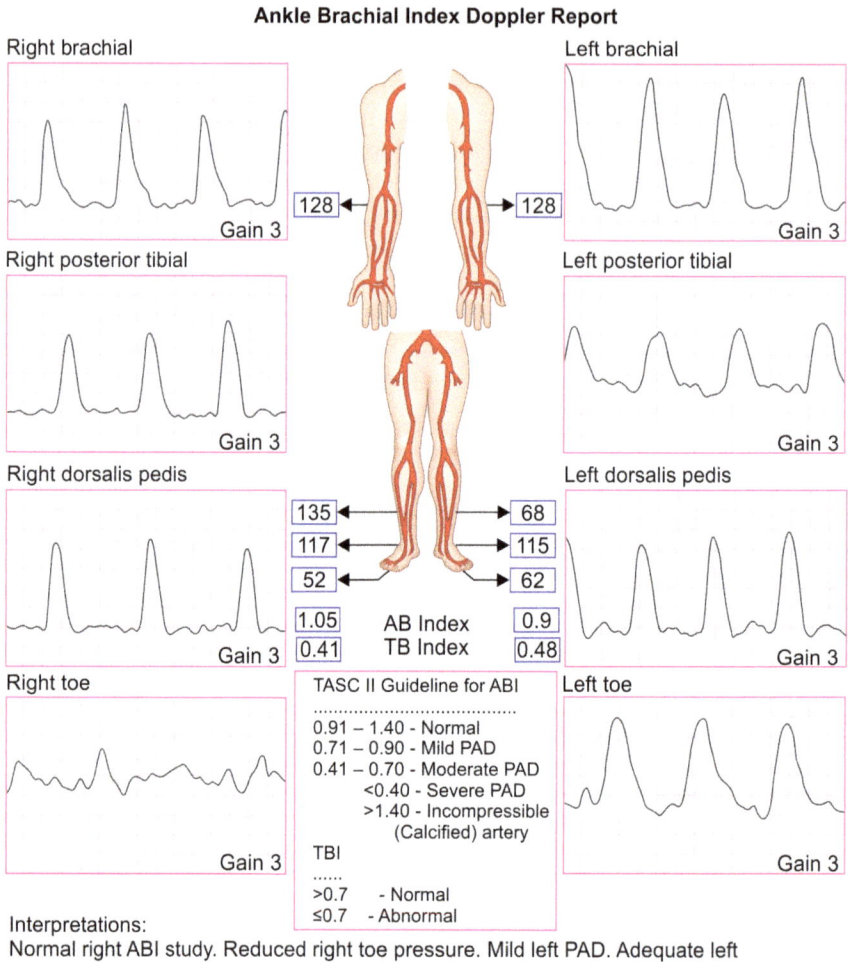

FIG. 1: Ankle brachial pressure index (ABPI), toe brachial index (TBI), and toe pressure (TP) in patient with diabetes and peripheral arterial disease.

with diabetes are highly variable (29-100% and 42-97%, respectively) (**Fig. 1**). TP measurements and TBI are useful in patients with diabetes due to the relative sparing of the digital arteries. TBI > 0.6 is predictive of tissue healing. Tissue perfusion can also be estimated by measuring the $TcPO_2$ with an electrode attached to the foot, which quantifies the transfer of oxygen molecules to the skin surface (**Table 1**), which helps in identifying patients with foot ulceration who are more likely to benefit from conservative management rather than revascularization.

Some other tests that have been used include pulse volume recording (PVR), photo plethysmography (PPG), and SPP.

TABLE 1: Summary of noninvasive laboratory investigation to assess perfusion status.[2]

Test	Normal	Mild disease	Moderate disease	Severe disease
ABPI	0.9–1.1	0.7–0.9	0.4–0.7	<0.4
TBI	>0.7	0.5–0.7	0.35–0.5	<0.35
TcPO$_2$ (mm Hg)	>40	20–40	20–40	<20
PVR	Triphasic	Biphasic	Biphasic	Monophasic
SPP (mm Hg)	>50	30–50	30–50	<30

(ABPI: ankle brachial pressure index; PVR: pulse wave recording waveforms; SPP: skin perfusion pressure; TBI: toe brachial index)

The National Institute for Health and Care Excellence in the UK recommends color duplex ultrasound (CDUS) imaging as the first line for all people being considered for revascularization. CDUS provides both anatomical details and physiological assessment of the blood flow at specific arterial sites. While CDUS has the advantage of being non-invasive and relatively inexpensive, it is hampered by diffuse segmental involvement, calcification and edema, in addition to its reliability being dependent on operator expertise. Intra-arterial DSA is still regarded as the best imaging modality. It not only provides high spatial resolution for planning revascularization, but also has the advantage of allowing endovascular intervention during the same procedure. The disadvantages of DSA include the use of an iodinated contrast medium that risks contrast-induced nephropathy in individuals with diabetes and renal insufficiency; it is an invasive procedure with potential complications from arterial puncture. Other less invasive modalities to image the arterial tree include computed tomography angiography (CTA) and contrast-enhanced magnetic resonance angiography (CE-MRA).

MANAGEMENT

Peripheral arterial disease is the most potent risk factor associated with failure of a DFU to heal. In addition to ischemia, other factors that affect the healing of DFU include poor glycemic control, infection, renal disease, microvascular dysfunction, poor collateral circulation and the presence of abnormal loading of the foot. Adverse wound healing of DFUs is related to the severity and extent of all these factors. Other factors that should be considered before the decision is made to revascularize include patient characteristics, comorbidities and life expectancy, as well as whether preservation of the limb would improve quality of life. People with diabetes, PAD and end-stage renal disease undergoing revascularization are one of the highest risk groups for perioperative mortality (5%). One year after operation, only 60% of these patients survived and only 70% still have their limb. Around 60% achieve wound healing at 1 year after revascularization, but 40% of these develop a new or recurrent ulcer within 12 months.

The International Working Group of the Diabetic Foot (IWGDF, an international consensus group in the management of people with diabetic foot disease) recommends an initial trial of non-operative management for people with a DFU where non-invasive vascular tests suggest that the perfusion is reasonable (indicated by one or more of the following ABPI > 0.6; $TcPO_2$ > 50 mm Hg; TP > 55 mm Hg). The IWGDF recommends the WIfI classification system to guide clinicians in estimating the 1 year risk of leg amputation and thus the potential benefit of revascularization for DFU. WIfI provides a more integrated wound overview by using a combination of scores for wound (based on depth of ulcer or extent of gangrene), ischemia (based on ankle pressure, TP, or $TcPO_2$), and foot infection (**Fig. 2**).

Ischemic ulcers should not be debrided until revascularization has been performed. While necrotic areas or frankly gangrenous digits will ultimately require

Score	Wound (W)	Ischemia (I)			Foot infection (FI)
		ABPI	AP	TP/$TcPO_2$	
0	No ulcer (ischemic rest pain)	>0.8	>100	>60	No infection
1	Small, shallow ulcer on distal leg or foot without gangrene	0.6–0.79	70–100	40–59	Local infection involving only skin/subcutaneous tissue
2	Deeper ulcer with exposed bone, joint or tendon ± gangrenous changes limited to toes	0.4–0.59	50–70	30–39	Local infection involving deeper than skin/subcutaneous tissue
3	Extensive deep ulcer, full thickness heel ulcer ± calcaneal involvement ± extensive gangrene	<0.4	<50	<30	Systemic inflammatory response syndrome

SVS WIfI clinical limb stage
Based on estimated risk of amputation at 1 year

	Ischemia - 0				Ischemia - 1				Ischemia - 2				Ischemia - 3			
W-0	1	1	2	3	1	2	3	4	2	2	3	4	2	3	3	4
W-1	1	1	2	3	1	2	3	4	2	3	4	4	3	3	4	4
W-2	2	2	3	4	3	3	4	4	3	4	4	4	4	4	4	4
W-3	3	3	4	4	4	4	4	4	4	4	4	4	4	4	4	4
	FI-0	FI-1	FI-2	FI-3	FI-0	FI-1	FI-2	FI-3	FI-0	FI-1	FI-2	FI-3	FI-0	FI-1	FI-2	FI-3

SVS WIfI clincal stage and 1-year rate of major amputations Weighted mean of published studies, n = 2,779 patients'		
Clinical stage 1	Very low risk	0.75%
Clinical stage 2	Low risk	5.9%
Clinical stage 3	Moderate risk	8.4%
Clinical stage 4	High risk	25%
Clinical stage 5 = Unsalvageable limb		

(ABPI: ankle brachial pressure index; AP: ankle pressure; TP: toe pressure; $TcPO_2$: transcutaneous oxygen pressure)

FIG. 2: Society for Vascular Surgery (SVS) wound, ischemia, foot infection (WIfI) classification.

some sort of amputation, this must be performed at a level where perfusion is adequate for healing. As long as there is no significant infection, debridement and amputation for dry necrosis should also be delayed until after revascularization.[3]

The indications for treating arterial occlusive disease in diabetics are similar to non-diabetic patients: Lifestyle limiting claudication, rest pain and tissue loss that is associated with non-healing ulcers and gangrenous changes.[4]

Treatment options in diabetic foot and PAD include the following:
- Medical therapy:
    - Optimization of comorbidities/risk factors
    - Supervised exercise therapy for claudicants
    - Antiplatelets drugs
    - Statin
    - Cessation of smoking or tobacco consumption in any form
- Surgery:
    - Endovascular interventions
    - Open surgical bypass
    - Amputation (minor/major)

SURGICAL OPTIONS OF TREATMENT

The aim of revascularization in patients with PAD is to achieve inline pulsatile flow to the foot by targeting the best vessel available. This can be direct revascularization or indirect revascularization based on the distal runoff. Angiosome-directed approach has been the favored approach of vascular surgeons. The angiosome concept was first described by Taylor and Palmer. The foot and ankle comprise six angiosomes, arising from three tibial vessels. Targeting revascularization of the vessel directly supplying the anatomical area of tissue loss should be more effective than restoring pulsatile blood flow through collateral vessels from neighboring angiosomes.[5] The prediction of patients most likely to require and to benefit from revascularization can be based on the SVS WIfI lower extremity threatened limb classification (**Fig. 2**).

There are no large scale randomized trials specifically comparing endovascular with surgical revascularization in people with diabetes, PAD and foot ulceration. The Bypass versus Angioplasty in Severe Ischemia of the Leg (BASIL) trial is often quoted as a guide to revascularization in the treatment of CLTI. Among the 452 patients randomized to bypass or endovascular intervention, perioperative morbidity was higher with surgery, but amputation-free and overall survivals were similar in both groups at 1 year. However, at the 2-year interval, surgery was associated with a reduced risk of amputation and death. The authors concluded that angioplasty should be used first for patients with a life expectancy of 2 or fewer years and that bypass is preferred when a vein conduit is available (**Fig. 3**).

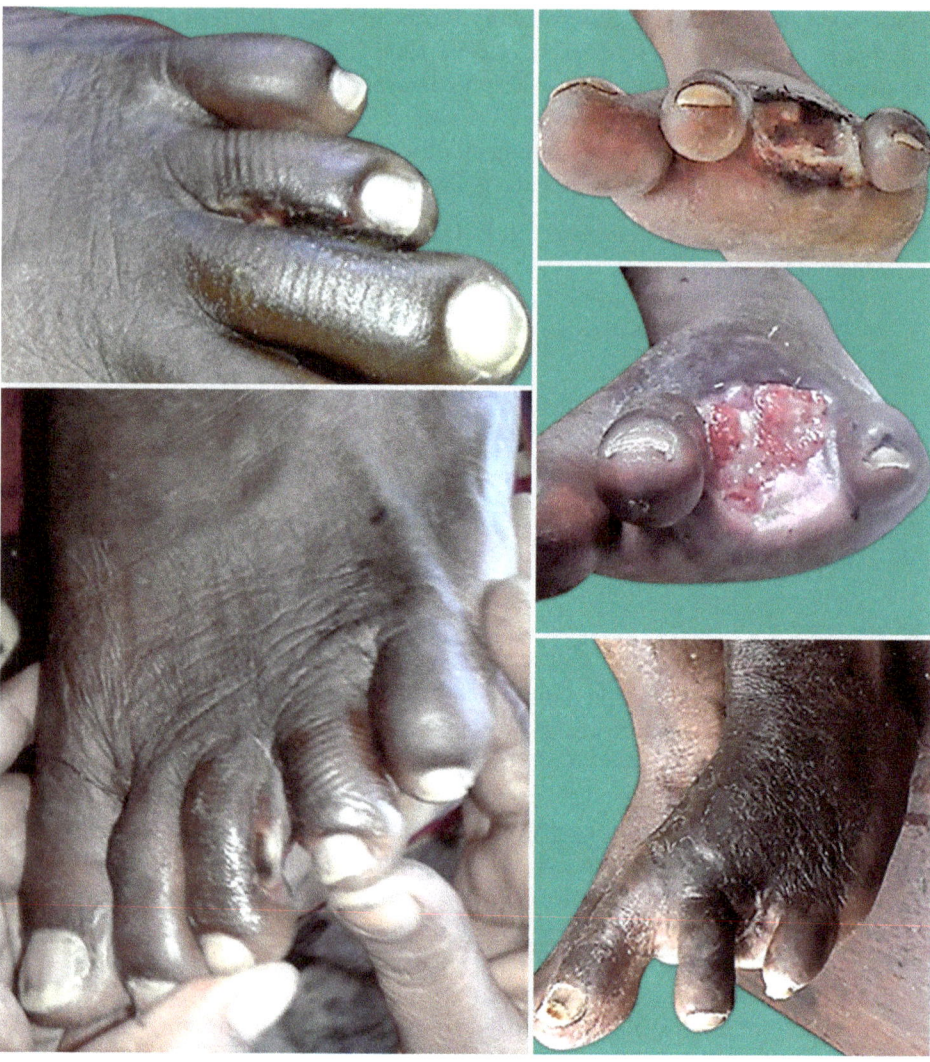

FIG. 3: 65-year-old lady with diabetes mellitus and interdigital ulcer, infection, and ischemia W1I3fI1. Wound healed completely after revascularization.

Although endovascular revascularization is done under local anesthesia and considered lower risk than bypass surgery, the IWGDF systematic review on the effectiveness of revascularization of the ulcerated diabetic foot in patients with PAD reported the perioperative mortality rate was similar following endovascular or open revascularization (both 2%). There is a higher reintervention rate following angioplasty. Surgical bypass with an autologous vein has better durability, but in

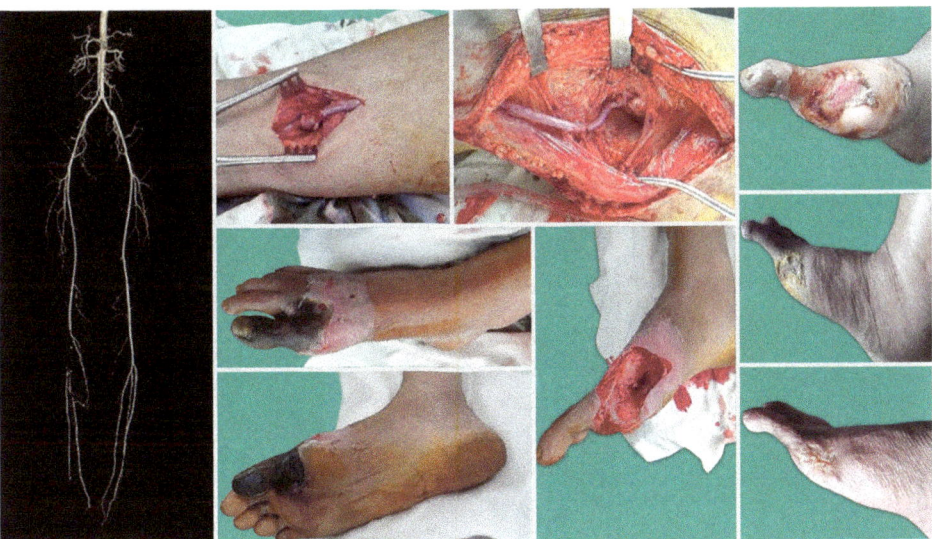

FIG. 4: 55-year-old lady with diabetes mellitus (DM) and gangrene W2I1fl1—wound completely healed after femoro-percutaneous transluminal angioplasty (PTA) bypass using vein conduit followed by great toe amputation.

patients with multiple comorbidities and a short life expectancy, an endovascular first approach to restoring perfusion may be justified.[6]

Restoration of foot perfusion in DFU is only part of the treatment and any revascularization procedure should be part of a multidisciplinary approach that also includes infection control, regular wound debridement, off-loading, glycemic control as well as treatment of comorbidities. This should be maintained, particularly after successful intervention (**Figs. 4** to **7**).

If there is extensive wet gangrene with overwhelming sepsis and ischemia, amputation is essential to save life.

The choice of intervention depends on the degree of ischemia, the extent of arterial disease, the extent of the wound, the presence or absence of infection and available expertise (**Flowchart 1**) (**Fig. 8**).

The recommendations of SVS are as follows:
- Patients with diabetes have ankle brachial index (ABI) measurements performed when they reach 50 years of age (grade 2C) and those with prior history of DFU, prior abnormal vascular examination, prior intervention for peripheral vascular disease, or known atherosclerotic cardiovascular disease (coronary, cerebral, or renal) have an annual vascular examination of lower extremities and feet including ABI and TPs (grade 2C).

- Patients with DFU have pedal perfusion assessed by ABI, ankle and pedal Doppler arterial waveforms, and either toe systolic pressure or TcPO$_2$ annually (grade 1B).
- Revascularization by surgical bypass or endovascular therapy (grade 1B).[7-10]

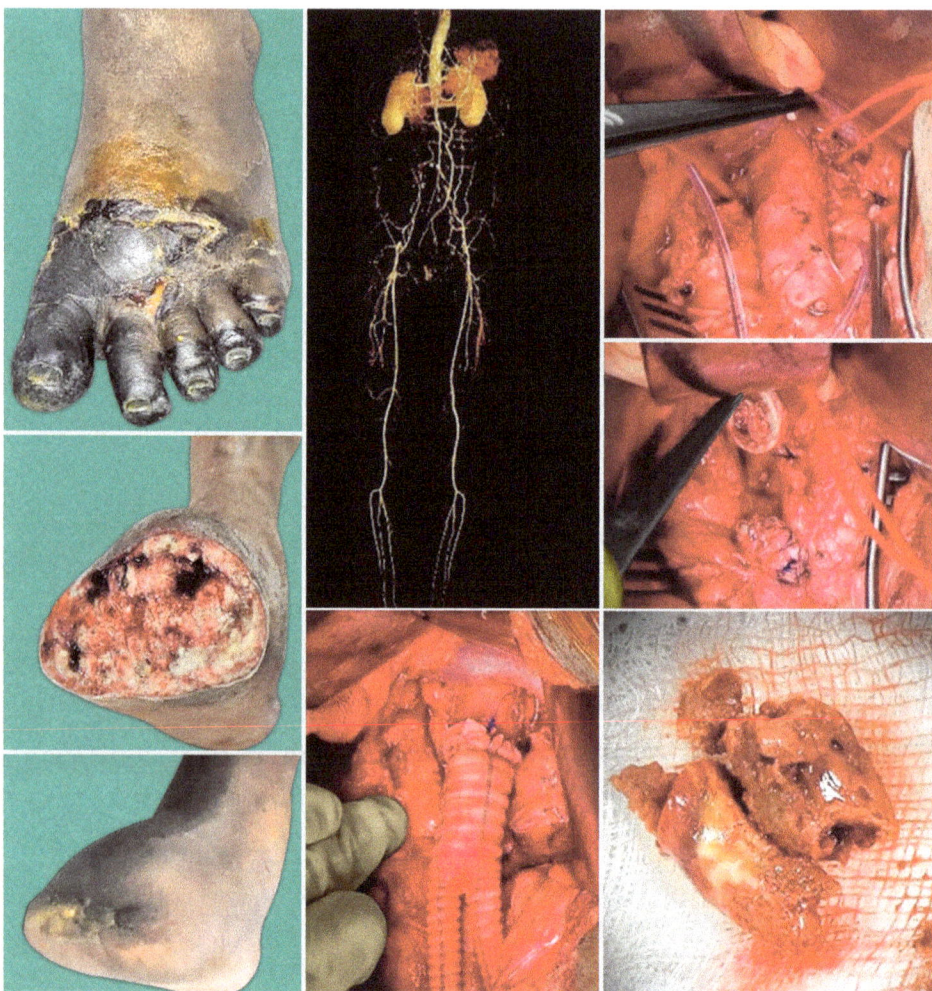

FIG. 5: 60-year-old presenting with extensive gangrene of the forefoot W3I3fl1—surgical revascularization done with aortobifemoral bypass and transmetatarsal amputation.

Peripheral Vascular Disease: Clinical Approach

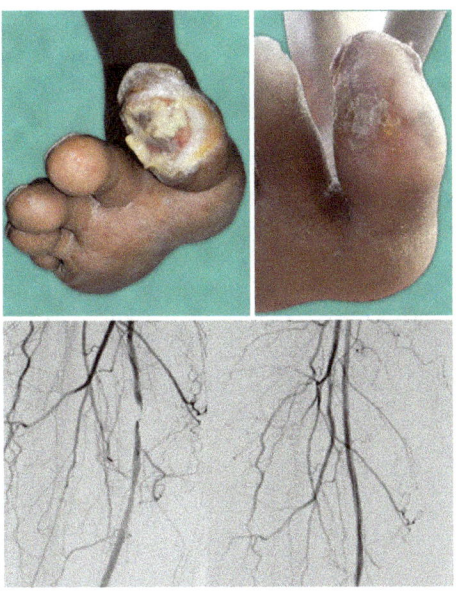

FIG. 6: 50-year-old having diabetes mellitus (DM), presenting with great toe ulcer W1I2fl0. Wound healed completely after percutaneous femoral angioplasty.

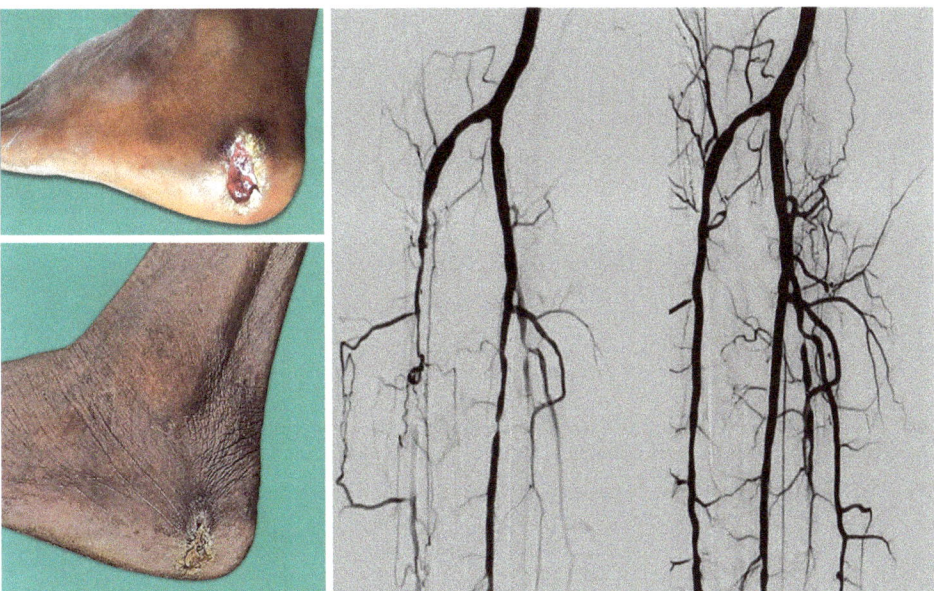

FIG. 7: 70-year-old gentleman who have diabetes mellitus (DM), presenting with a heel ulcer W1I2fl0. Lower picture should provide ulcer status after tibial angioplasty.

Peripheral Vascular Disease: Clinical Approach

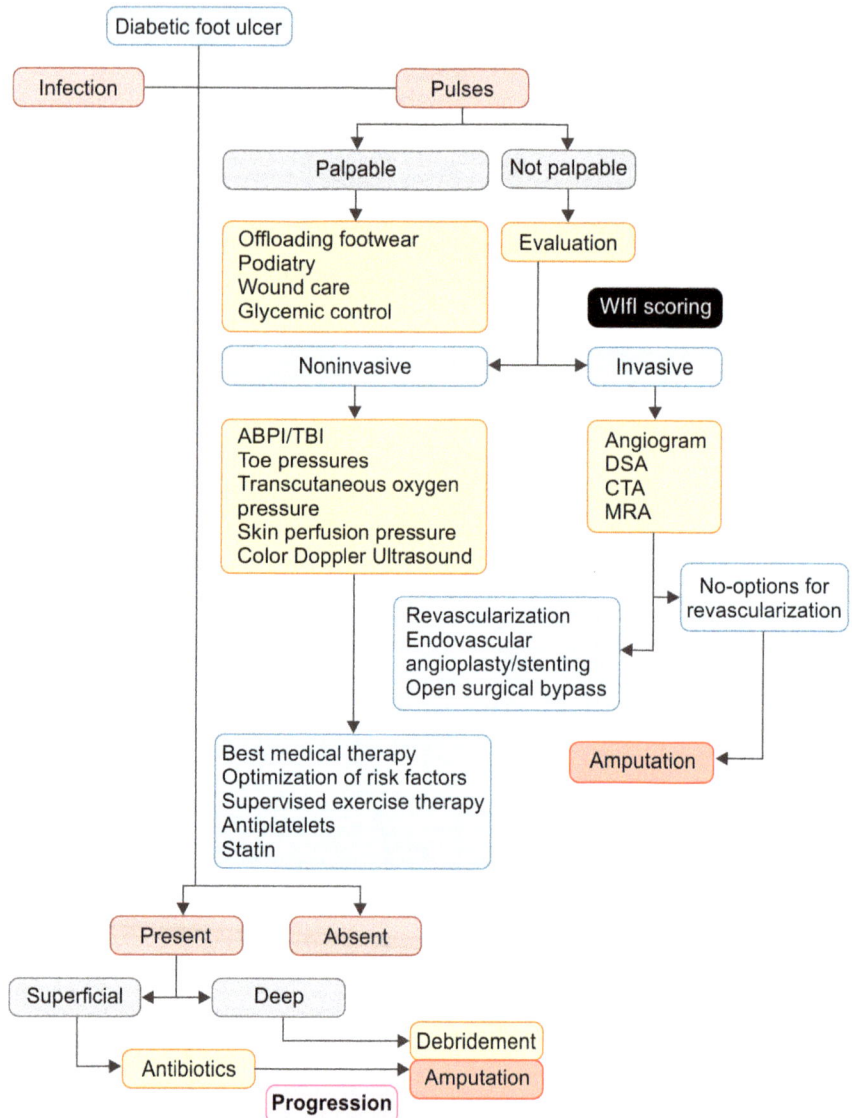

(ABPI: ankle-brachial pressure index; CTA: computed tomography angiogram; DSA: digital subtraction angiography; MRA: magnetic resonance angiogram; TBI: toe-brachial index; WIfI: wound, ischemia, foot infection)

FLOWCHART 1: Algorithm for patients with peripheral arterial disease.

Peripheral Vascular Disease: Clinical Approach

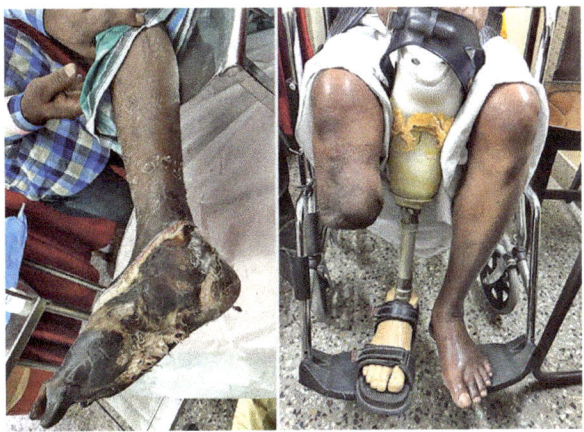

FIG. 8: 65-year-old presenting with extensive gangrene in sepsis W3I2fI3 (clinical stage 4) requiring a below knee amputation.

CONCLUSION

Peripheral arterial disease is common among patients with DM. A simple bedside examination helps in identifying these patients. If the patients have reduced peripheral pulses, they should undergo an ABPI, thereby confirming the evidence of vascular compromise. Further invasive investigations such as CTA, MRA or DSA helps in localizing the areas of the vascular compromise and in treating them appropriately. Hence, an early diagnosis of PAD helps to prevent future gangrene as well as much-dreaded amputations.

REFERENCES

1. Hinchliffe RJ, Forsythe RO, Apelqvist J, Boyko EJ, Fitridge R, Hong JP, et al. Guidelines on diagnosis, prognosis, and management of peripheral artery disease in patients with foot ulcers and diabetes (IWGDF 2019 update). Diabetes Metab Res Rev. 2020;36 Suppl 1:e3276.
2. Mills JL, Conte MS, Armstrong DG, Pomposelli FB, Schanzer A, Sidawy AN, et al. The Society for Vascular Surgery Lower Extremity Threatened Limb Classification System: Risk stratification based on Wound, Ischemia, and foot Infection (WIfI). J Vasc Surg. 2014;59(1):220-34.e2.
3. Hingorani A, LaMuraglia GM, Henke P, Meissner MH, Loretz L, Zinszer KM, et al. The management of diabetic foot: A clinical practice guideline by the Society for Vascular Surgery in collaboration with the American Podiatric Medical Association and the Society for Vascular Medicine. J Vasc Surg. 2016;63(2):3S-21S.
4. Mills JL. The application of the Society for Vascular Surgery Wound, Ischemia, and foot Infection (WIfI) classification to stratify amputation risk. J Vasc Surg. 2017;65(3):591-3.
5. Lepäntalo M, Apelqvist J, Setacci C, Ricco JB, de Donato G, Becker F, et al. Chapter V: Diabetic Foot. Eur J Vasc Endovasc Surg. 2011;42 Suppl 2:S60-74.
6. Brownrigg JRW, Apelqvist J, Bakker K, Schaper NC, Hinchliffe RJ. Evidence-based Management of PAD & the Diabetic Foot. Eur J Vasc Endovasc Surg. 2013;45(6):673-81.

7. Ricco J-B, Bartelink M-LEL, Björck M, Brodmann M, Cohnert T, Collet JP, et al. Document covering atherosclerotic disease of extracranial carotid and vertebral, mesenteric, renal, upper and lower extremity arteries Endorsed by: the European Stroke Organization (ESO). Eur Heart J. 2018;39(9):763-816.
8. Bradbury AW, Adam DJ, Bell J, Forbes JF, Fowkes FGR, Gillespie I, et al. Bypass versus Angioplasty in Severe Ischaemia of the Leg (BASIL) trial: Analysis of amputation free and overall survival by treatment received. J Vasc Surg. 2010;51(5 Suppl):18S-31S.
9. Forsythe RO, Apelqvist J, Boyko EJ, Fitridge R, Hong JP, Katsanos K, et al. Effectiveness of revascularisation of the ulcerated foot in patients with diabetes and peripheral artery disease: A systematic review. Diabetes Metab Res Rev. 2020;36 Suppl 1:e3279.
10. Humphries MD, Brunson A, Hedayati N, Romano P, Melnkow J. Amputation risk in patients with diabetes mellitus and peripheral artery disease using statewide data. Ann Vasc Surg. 2016;30: 123-31.

PRAMOD KARAN SETHI

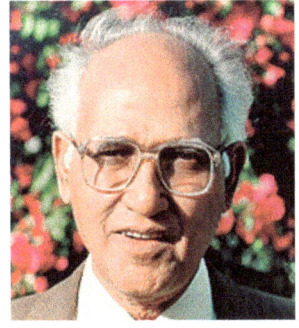

Pramod Karan Sethi was the coinventor of the Jaipur foot. He was born on November 23, 1927, in Varanasi, India. He was working as an orthopedic surgeon at Sawai Man Singh Hospital in Jaipur in the late 60s. He worked with individuals who required rehabilitation and found that the rural populace often abandoned the available prosthesis which led to rigidity and limited mobility in them. Prostheses from the West were expensive and not suitable for performing agricultural work barefoot. Along with Ram Chandra, a craftsman providing vocational training to patients with leprosy, Sethi attempted to design a form of artificial limb more suited to the Indian population, known as the "Jaipur Foot". The Bhagwan Mahaveer Viklang Sahayata Samiti (BMVSS), a Jaipur charity, has fitted over 3 lakh amputees for the Jaipur Foot for free. Sethi was awarded the Padma Shri by the Government of India in 1981 and was elected a fellow of the British Royal College of Surgeons.

Footwear and Offloading Aids in Diabetic Foot

Bobeena Rachel Chandy, Naveen Cherian Thomas

INTRODUCTION

The presence of diabetic foot indicates an abnormality of physiological functioning by and large related to neurological dysfunction due to chronic, uncontrolled blood glucose levels. The degree of neuropathy may vary but the resultant complication, namely the ulcers, are the most common non-traumatic cause for lower limb amputations. Clinical evidence shows that proper footwear and therapeutic orthotics help in prevention of amputations and deformities, by protecting the insensate foot from unnoticed trauma and excessive plantar pressures that occur during ambulation.

As awareness of diabetic foot disease and non-healing ulcers leading to amputations increases among the diabetic population, the need to know about new possibilities for the prevention and management among medical personnel has become essential.[1]

PRINCIPLES OF MANAGEMENT

The lifetime risk of a person with DM to develop foot ulcer is estimated to be 15–25%. The annual risk of developing DFU in patients with DM is estimated to be about 2% and is expected to increase to 17–60% over the next 3 years, in those patients with previous history of foot ulceration.

With the knowledge that most amputations in patient with DM are preceded by ulceration, it is paramount that footcare protocols are developed for prevention and care.[2]

As per the International Working Group on the Diabetic Foot (IWGDF) Guidance 2019 document, the Evidence-based International Consensus Guidance puts down five key elements that underpin prevention of foot problems:
- Identification of the at-risk foot
- Regular inspection and examination of the at-risk foot
- Education of patient, family, and healthcare providers
- Routine use of appropriate footwear
- Treatment of pre-ulcerative signs

TABLE 1: The International Working Group on the Diabetic Foot (IWGDF) risk classification system 2019 and preventative screening frequency.[4]

Category	Characteristics	Frequency
0	No peripheral neuropathy	Once a year
1	Peripheral neuropathy	Once every 6 months
2	Peripheral neuropathy with peripheral artery disease and/or a foot deformity	Once every 3–6 months
3	Peripheral neuropathy and a history of foot ulcer or lower extremity amputation	Once every 1–3 months

According to the guidance consensus, healthcare providers should follow a standardized and consistent strategy for evaluating a DFU, as this will guide further evaluation and therapy (**Table 1**). The following items must be addressed: Type, cause, site and depth, and signs of infection. The seven key elements that underpin DFU treatment are:
1. Relief of pressure and protection of the ulcer
2. Restoration of skin perfusion
3. Treatment of infection
4. Metabolic control and treatment of other comorbidities
5. Local wound care
6. Education for patient and relatives; and
7. Prevention of recurrence[3]

CASE SCENARIOS

Case 1

A 50-year-old gentleman, known to have type 2 diabetes mellitus (T2DM) over the last 4 years, presented to the integrated diabetic foot clinic with concerns of a non-healing ulcer over the plantar aspect of the left big toe for a 3-month duration. He gave history of trauma due to a sharp pebble, while walking barefoot in the field, prior to the onset of the ulcer.

On Examination (Figs. 1A to C)

A (1 × 1) cm ulcer over the plantar aspect of left greater toe with surrounding callosity. There was diffuse swelling surrounding the ulcer. Depth of the ulcer was 0.5 cm and there was no discharge. All peripheral pulses were well felt. He was using a worn-out microcellular rubber (MCR) footwear with back strap at that time.

Intervention

Parring of the callosity was done in the first visit, and he was prescribed new *MCR footwear with anterior rocker* (**Figs. 1F** and **G**). Daily saline dressings with strict

Footwear and Offloading Aids in Diabetic Foot

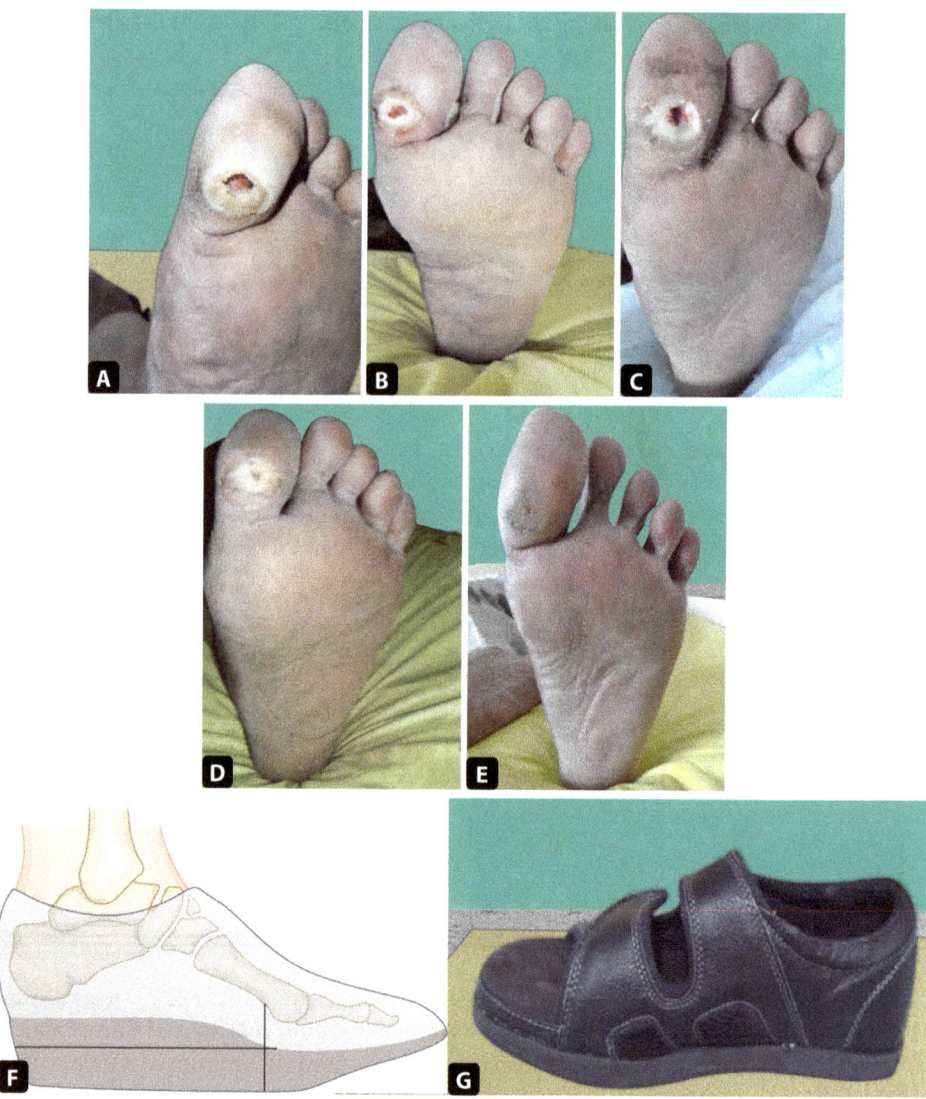

FIGS. 1A TO G: (A) 1 × 1 cm ulcer over the plantar aspect of left greater toe with surrounding callosity; (B) Ulcer bed exposed following debridement of the surrounding callosity; (C) Two weekly review follow ups, size of the ulcer was reduced; (D and E) Review visits, ulcer completely healed; (F) Footwear with anterior rocker bottom; (G) Microcellular rubber footwear with anterior rocker bottom.

glycemic control and adherence to foot care was advised. He came to the clinic for review once in 2 weeks and the ulcer was noted to have completely healed in 3 months' time (**Figs. 1D** and **E**).

Anterior rocker bottom for diabetic footwear helps by minimizing the duration of loading the forefoot during the push off phase of the gait cycle. A 10–15° angulation is given for the rocker effect to happen.

Case 2

55-year-old Mr B, known to have T2DM (poorly controlled) since 18 years, hypertension for 14 years and coronary artery disease, postcoronary artery bypass graft (CABG) in 2012, underwent first ray amputation of the left big toe for cellulitis. The surgical wound was not sutured, and the wound left open to heal by secondary intention. He was referred to the integrated diabetic foot clinic for offloading and management of postoperative wound.

On Examination (Fig. 2A)

A (4 × 5) cm ulcer over the distal medial aspect of left foot with healthy granulation issue at the base of the ulcer. There was no significant discharge from the wound. Peripheral pulses were felt.

Intervention

The patient was given the choice of total contact casting (TCC) with Bohler iron (**Figs. 2B** to **F**) for complete offloading. However, he wanted to have a trial of healing without the intervention. Therefore, he was advised daily dressing and limited mobility with a walker. At review in 2 weeks, there was no significant changes in the size of the ulcer, therefore, the patient requested to be put on a TCC with a Bohler iron. This was was applied with the plaster ending at the level of the midfoot to allow for daily dressings. The cast was changed every 2 weeks and at the end of 2 months, the wound had completely healed.

Case 3

53-year-old Mr. C, known to have T2DM for the last 5 years, presented to the integrated diabetes foot clinic with a non-healing ulcer on the plantar surface of the left hindfoot with pus discharge for the last 2–3 weeks. There was no history of fever. He is known to have poorly controlled blood sugars.

On Examination (Fig. 3A)

A (3 × 0.5) cm ulcer over the plantar aspect of the left hindfoot with foul-smelling pus discharge was noted. The surrounding skin was warm and swollen, with an area of necrotic tissue. Peripheral pulses were well felt. His vital signs were normal.

Intervention

The ulcer was debrided and the pus was completely drained. A thorough wound wash was given with hydrogen peroxide and saline. The floor of the ulcer was exposed and daily saline dressings with complete offloading with use of crutches for mobility was advised. Medications were titrated for good glycemic control and he was also started on broad-spectrum antibiotics (in view of cellulitis) following a pus culture. The next review a week later showed healthy granulation tissue at the base of the ulcer. A *TCC with a Bohler iron* (**Figs. 3B** to **E**) for complete offloading was applied. A window was made over the ulcer for daily dressings; it healed over a period of 6 weeks. Thereafter, he was given MCR footwear. Footcare education was reinforced.

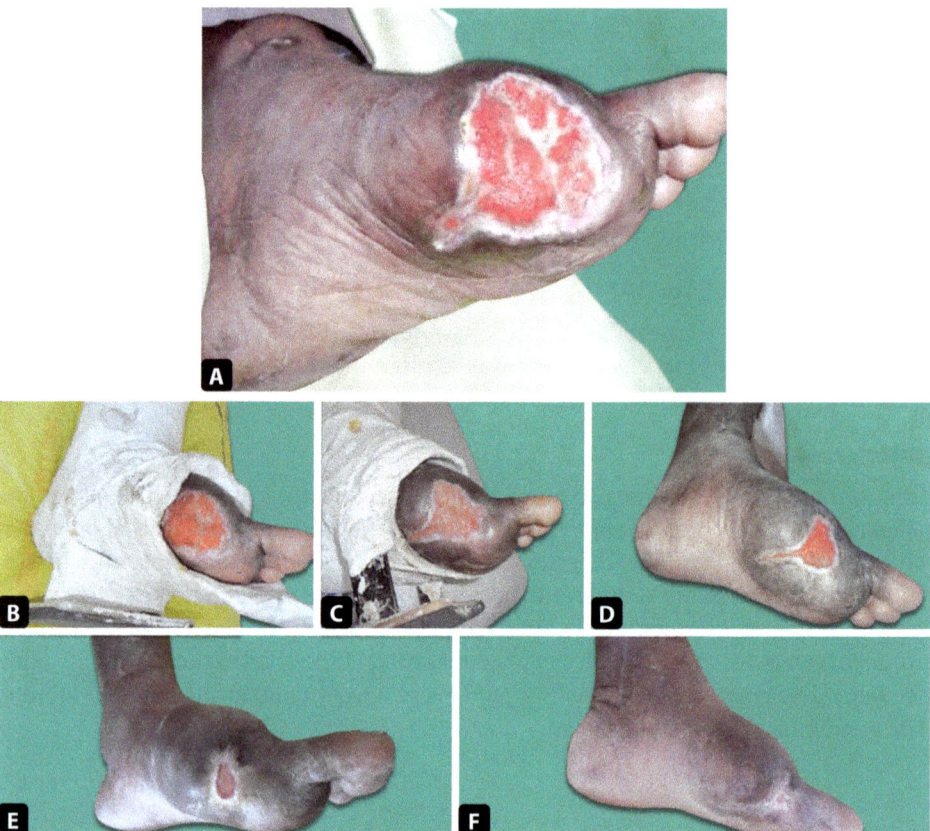

FIGS. 2A TO F: (A) 4 × 5 cm clean ulcer over the distal medial aspect of foot; (B) Bohler iron casting with the ulcer area exposed for daily dressing; (C) Ulcer size reduced after 1 week; (D and E) Weekly follow-up; (F) Ulcer completely healed at the end of 2 months.

A *Bohler iron* is an orthotic device which is used for complete offloading for plantar ulcers. The device has iron bars which go onto the sides of the cast and fixed with a proximal clamp. The bars are widened at the level of the malleoli to accommodate the natural curvatures of the casted limb. A layer of plaster of Paris is applied to the iron bars and the clamp to firmly anchor the orthosis to the below-knee cast, a layer of plaster of Paris is applied to the clamp and the iron bars. To the distal aspect of the iron bar, a supporting platform made of iron and a rubber sole is attached. This facilitates stability and weight-bearing during ambulation. An approximately two-finger breadth clearance is to be maintained between the heel and the platform. The window is cut out in the cast at the location of the plantar ulcer to leave it open for inspection and wound care. However, making a window for wound care is optional and at the discretion of the treating physician. A compensatory raise of the sole is given for the shoe of the contralateral foot.

Footwear and Offloading Aids in Diabetic Foot

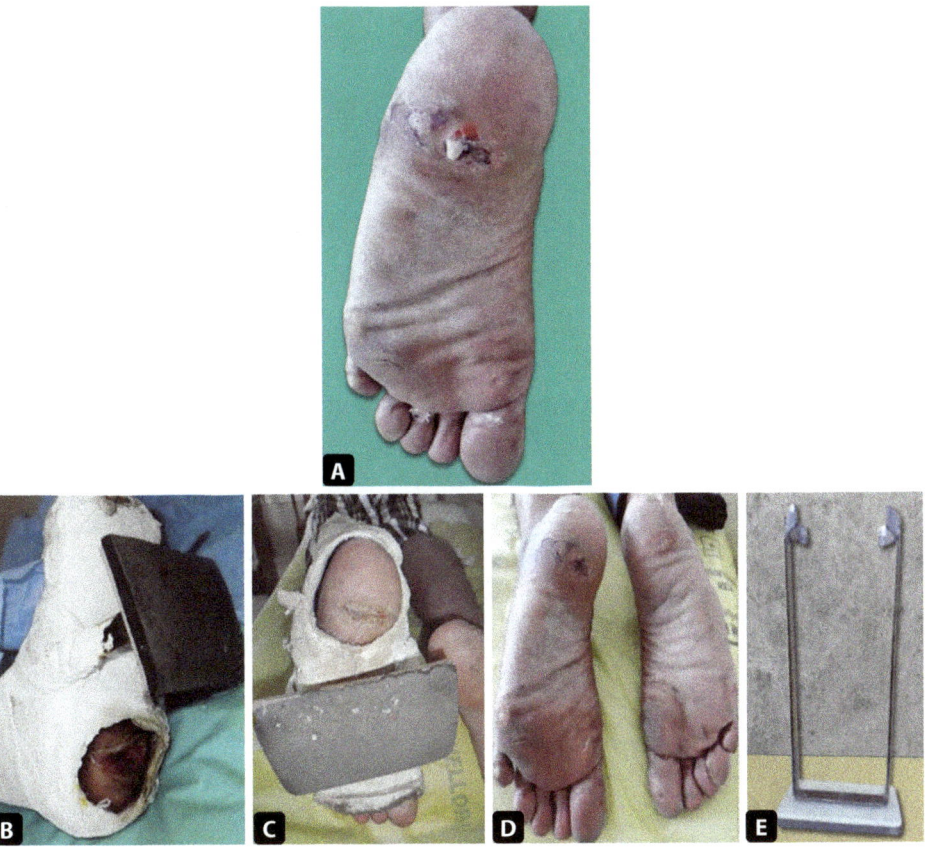

FIGS. 3A TO E: (A) Ulcer with pus discharge from the hindfoot; (B) Following the debridement of the ulcer, he was put a Bohler iron cast with a window made over the ulcer area for daily dressing; (C) After 4 weeks; (D) Ulcer completely healed after 6 weeks; (E) Bohler iron.

Case 4

A 50-year-old gentleman, known to have T2DM (uncontrolled) over a 10 year duration with diabetic neuropathy, systemic hypertension and dyslipidemia was referred to the integrated diabetic foot clinic with a deformity of the left foot and a non-healing chronic ulcer over the plantar aspect of the midfoot.

On Examination (Figs. 4A and B)

A (3 × 3) cm ulcer over the plantar aspect of the left midfoot, thickened skin, and hyperpigmentation was present in the area surrounding the ulcer. There was collapse of the medial arch of the foot. The base of the ulcer was clean and had granulation tissue. There was serous discharge from the wound. The left dorsalis pedis was feeble, but other pulses were well felt. His X-ray showed features of Charcot foot, grades 2–5 (**Figs. 4C** and **D**).

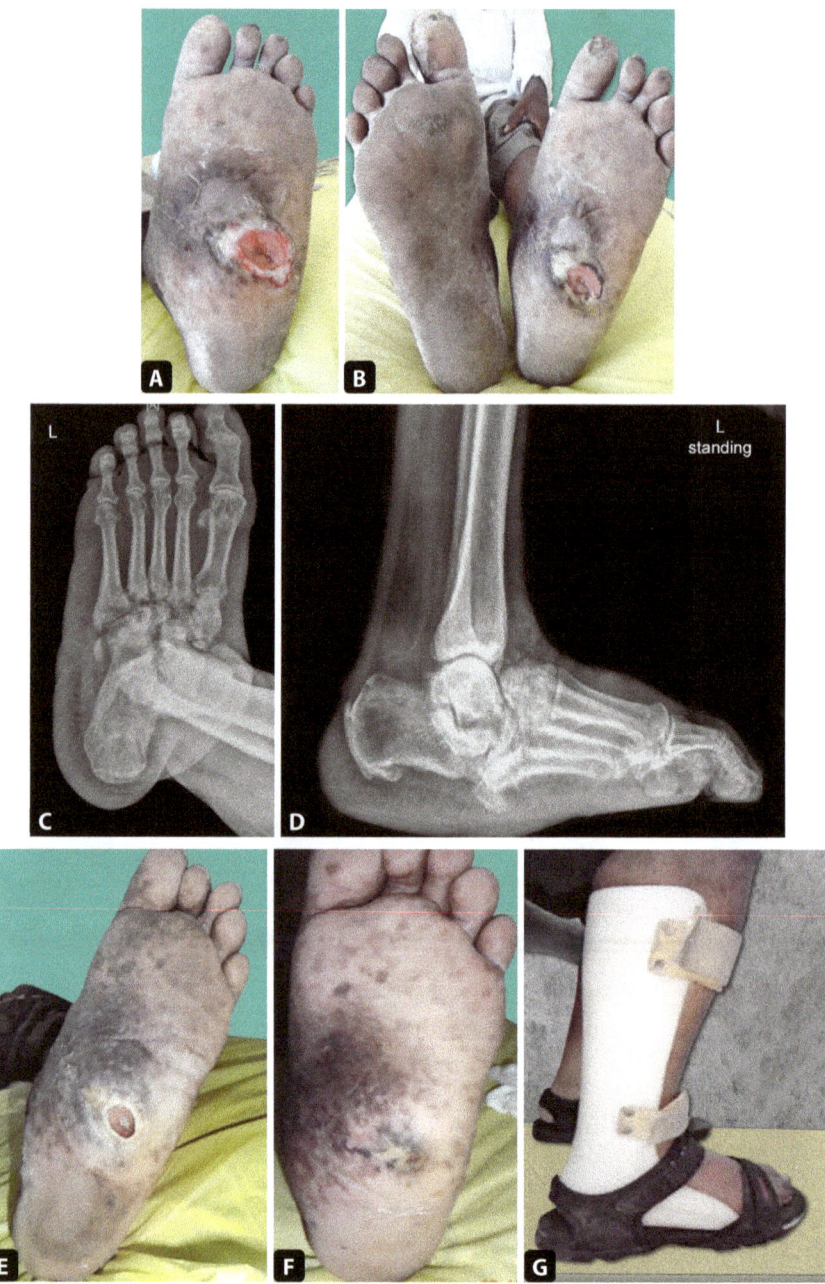

FIGS. 4A TO G: (A) Midfoot ulcer in the left foot plantar aspect, with surrounding callosities and hyperpigmentation; (B) Loss of medial arch of the foot (left), there is hyperpigmentation and callosity around the ulcer; (C and D) X-ray showing Charcot foot left side, chronic osteomyelitic changes over the tarsometatarsal joints, and loss of the medial arch; (E and F) Weekly reviews, after 6 weeks the ulcer is completely healed; (G) Ankle foot orthosis.

Intervention

A Serial TCC was fixed until the ulcer completely healed. Following this, he was prescribed a *left ankle foot orthosis (AFO) with MCR footwear* (**Figs. 4E** to **G**). He was referred to the vascular surgeons, thereafter.

An Ankle foot orthosis is a device used in those with DM and foot deformity as a result of Charcot's arthropathy, to maintain the foot architecture and prevent worsening of the deformity. It is also used for persons with a foot drop for mediolateral support and prevention of a foot slap.

Case 5

A 38-year-old Mr E, with young-onset T2DM (well controlled) for the last 7 years, presented to the integrated diabetes foot clinic with complaints of left foot pain and swelling over 4 months. There were no ulcers, calluses or fissures.

On Examination (Fig. 5A)

He was afebrile; the left foot was warm with diffuse edema up to ankle. The sole of the foot looked shiny and red. There was no break in the continuity of the skin. Peripheral pulses were felt.

Intervention

He was diagnosed to have acute Charcot arthropathy based on the clinical features and X-ray findings (**Figs. 5B** and **C**). He was advised complete offloading and crutch walking for 2 weeks, following which, a pneumatic boot was prescribed for 6 weeks (**Figs. 5D** and **E**). Long-term, he has been given a hinged (allowing 10° of dorsiflexion and plantar flexion) AFO to maintain the foot architecture and to allow for movements at the ankle.

Case 6

A 45-year-old gentleman, known to have T2DM for the last 10 years, presented to the integrated diabetic foot clinic with complaints of deformity of the right foot for 6 months with swelling and pain since 3 months.

On Examination (Figs. 6A and B)

There was diffuse swelling of the right foot upto the level of the ankle which was associated with warmth, valgus deformity of ankle along with forefoot abduction. The skin over the foot looked shiny and hyperpigmented when compared to the right foot. Peripheral pulses were well felt. An X-ray of the right foot showed destruction of the tarsometatarsal joints and diffuse osteopenia suggestive of Charcot foot, grades 3–5 (**Figs. 6C** and **D**).

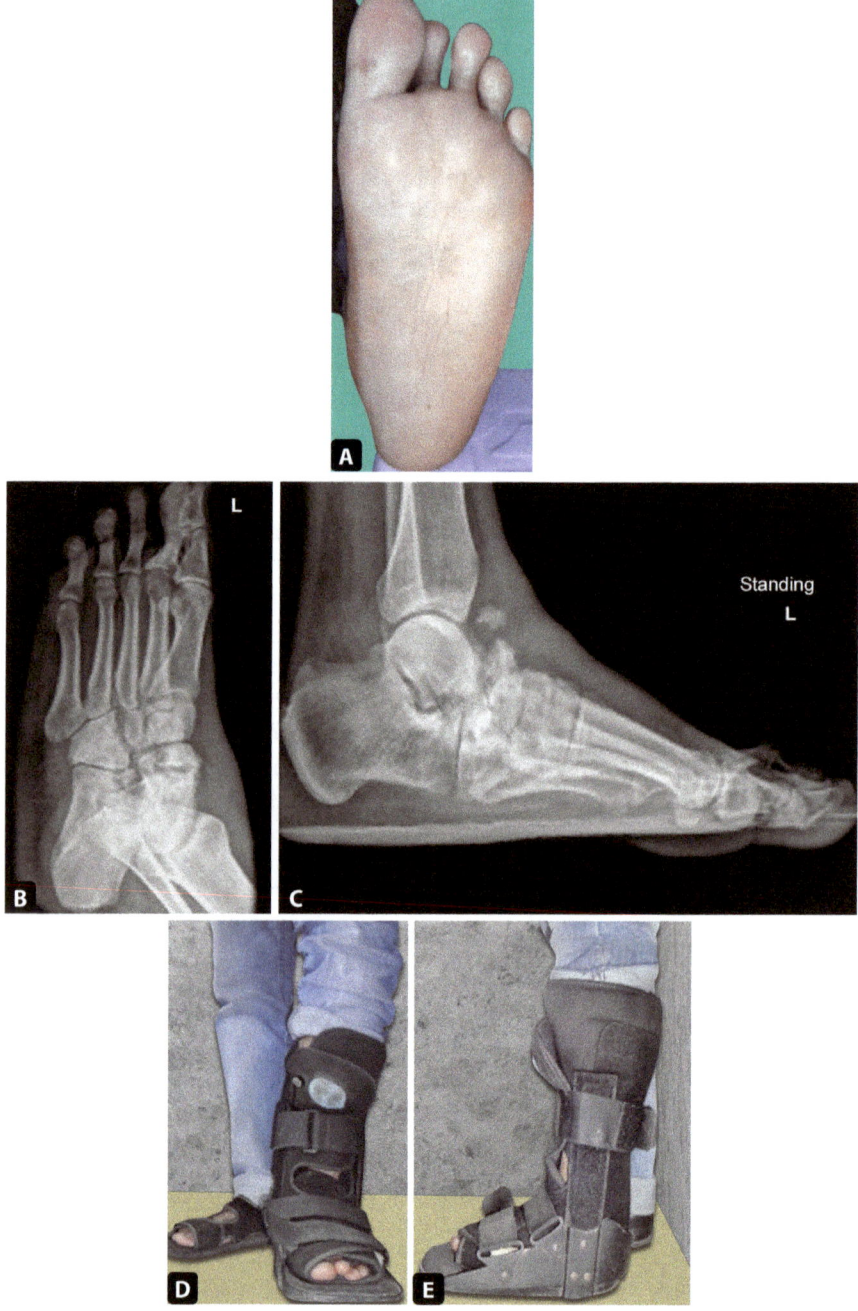

FIGS. 5A TO E: (A) Sole of the foot looking shiny, reddish, and edematous; (B and C) X-ray of the left foot showing features of Charcot arthropathy; (D and E) Pneumatic boot.

Intervention

He was prescribed a *patellar tendon-bearing ankle foot orthosis (PTB-AFO)* (**Fig. 6E**). A patellar tendon-bearing (PTB) orthosis is a custom molded plastic brace with an anterior shell attached to an AFO. The anterior shell is molded to take the contours

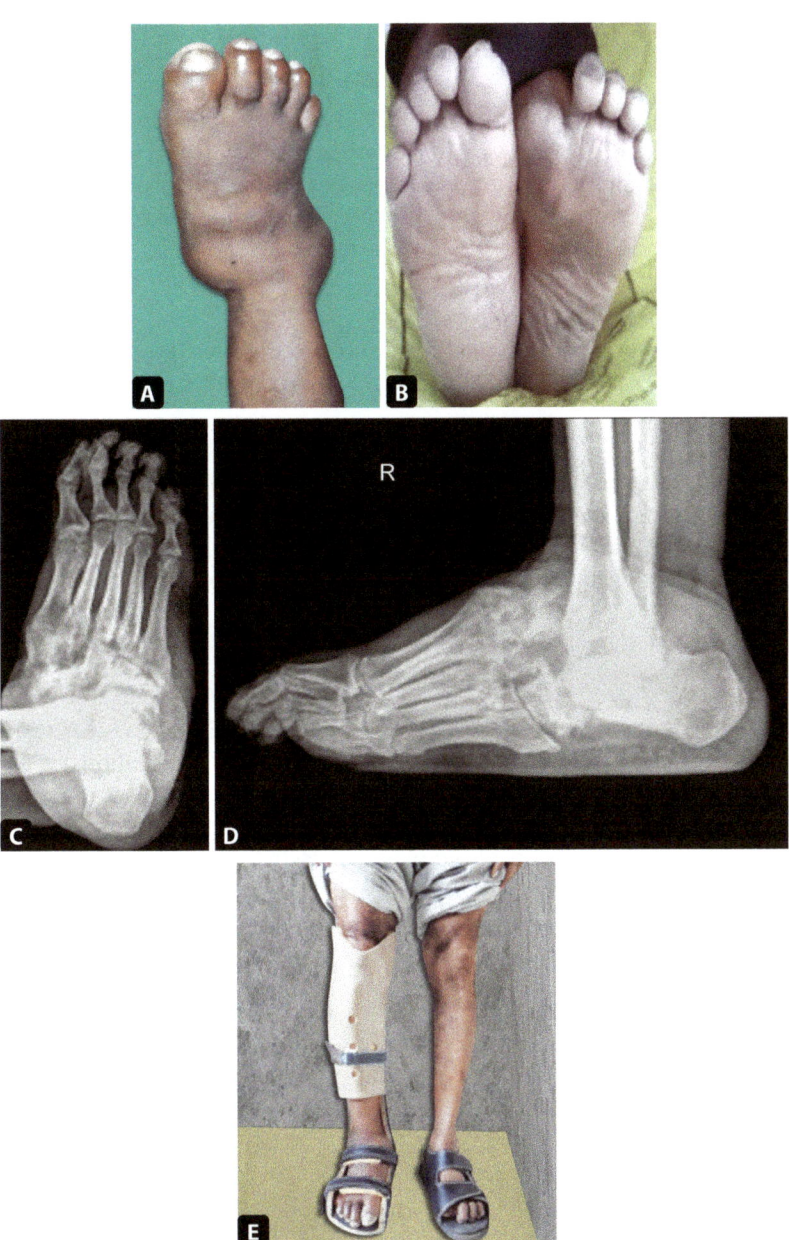

FIGS. 6A TO E: (A and B) Diffuse swelling of right foot, varus deformity of the ankle, and hyperpigmented skin; (C and D) X-ray of the right foot anteroposterior and lateral—destruction of tarsometatarsal joints and diffuse osteopenia; (E) Patellar tendon-bearing ankle foot orthosis.

of the patellar tendon at the knee. It redistributes the weight borne by the distal joint to the patellar tendon, thereby giving relief to the painful ankle and foot. It is given to persons with Charcot arthropathy for managing pain and may also be given for long-term management of Charcot's arthropathy for protecting the architecture of the foot by redistribution of load.

Case 7

A 55-year-old gentleman, known to have T2DM and hypertension for the last 15 years, was referred to the integrated foot clinic by surgeons following a forefoot amputation due to a preceding gangrene. The wound was not primarily closed and left to heal by secondary intention. The patient was a grocery shop owner in a rural area and had to work as he was the sole bread-winner for the family.

On Examination (Fig. 7A)

The ulcer had a clean base with healthy granulation tissue. There was no significant discharge from the wound. Blood sugars were well-controlled.

Intervention

As the patient was not willing for a total contact cast, he was prescribed a PTBO (**Fig. 7B**). He was advised to review in the clinic every 2 weeks. The ulcer completely healed in 8 weeks, following which he was given a foot prosthesis. Foot care was reinforced at every visit. He continued working and ambulating using the orthosis and crutches.

Case 8

A 68-year-old gentleman was seen in the integrated foot clinic for recurring ulcers on the distal aspect of the left residual limb. He had a forefoot amputation 3 years ago on the left side and fourth ray amputation on the right side. He lived a sedentary lifestyle and did not use any foot wear. He is a known diabetic with poorly controlled sugars, peripheral neuropathy and chronic smoker with ischemic heart disease.

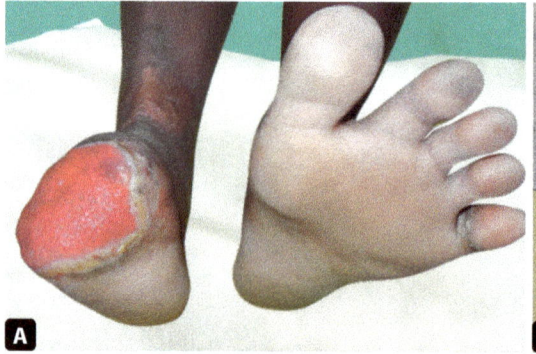
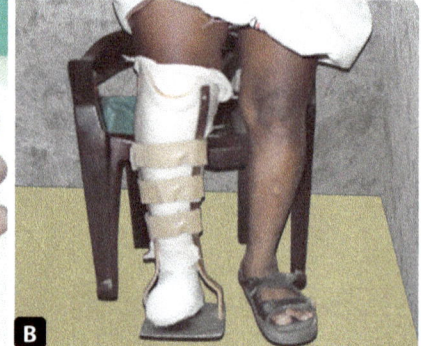

FIGS. 7A AND B: (A) Raw wound after a forefoot amputation; (B) Patellar tendon-bearing orthosis.

On Examination (Fig. 8A)

He had an eschar over the distal aspect of the residual limb. The foot was in equinus due to contracture of the tendo-Achilles. The anterior tibial artery was feeble on the left side on evaluation with a hand-held Doppler.

Intervention

This gentleman was admitted to the ward. Medical management for controlling blood glucose level was initiated. The wound underwent serial debridement and daily dressings till healthy granulation tissue was seen. A tendo-Achilles lengthening procedure was done to correct the equinus deformity which was the cause for the recurrent ulceration of the insensate foot. The foot was in a plaster cast (TCC) for 4 weeks following which he was given a prosthesis maintaining the foot in neutral and cosmetic forefoot (**Figs. 8B** and **C**).

Case 9

A 53-year-old lady was seen in in the integrated foot clinic for pain and redness over the left medial aspect of the first metatarsal head. She was recently diagnosed to have DM with fairly well-controlled glucose levels.

On Examination (Fig. 9)

She had a hallux valgus on the left side with a bunion. The skin over the bunion was inflamed with an impending ulcer.

Intervention

She was advised limited mobility and rest with foot end elevation. Anti-inflammatories and antibiotics were given. A readymade *silicone bunion shield* was prescribed for protection of the skin along with the use of MCR footwear.

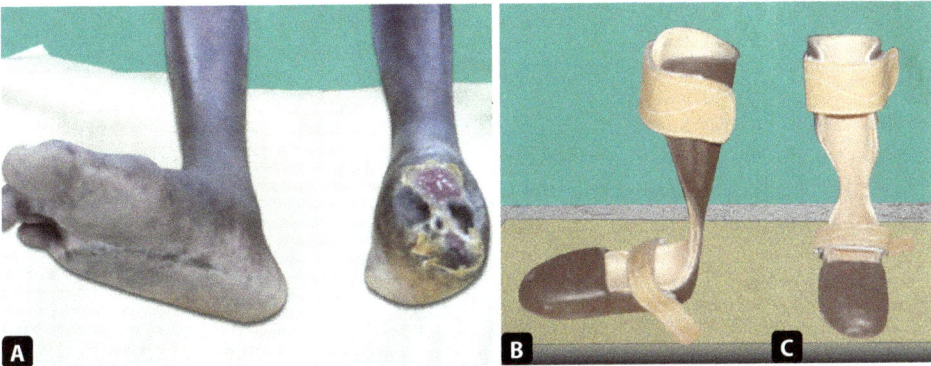

FIGS. 8A TO C: (A) Eschar over the distal aspect of the residual limb (left) with an equinus deformity; (B and C) Prosthesis for mid-foot amputation. The ankle and leg extension has been given to maintain the ankle in neutral and prevent further worsening of the equinus deformity.

Footwear and Offloading Aids in Diabetic Foot

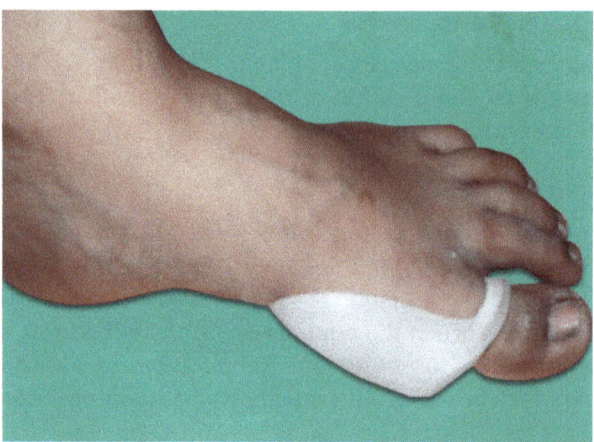

FIG. 9: Bunion shield.

Case 10

A 60-year-old temple priest was referred to the integrated clinic with a history of chronic callosities over the lateral aspect of the foot and ankle. He is known to have T2DM with fairly well-controlled glucose. There were no other complaints.

On Examination (Fig. 10)

He had callosities over the lateral malleoli and fifth metatarsal heads bilaterally. There were no other abnormalities. The peripheral pulsations were well-felt.

Intervention

The callosities were parred after foot soak in water. The patient was advised to strictly avoid cross-legged sitting. Footcare education was given and MCR footwear were prescribed.

Case 11

A 45-year-old lady was seen in the diabetes clinic for regular review. At the time, it was noted that she wore toe rings (**Fig. 11A**). She was advised to remove the toe rings by the diabetes educator. She presented to the integrated foot clinic, 3 months later with painful and swollen third toe.

On Examination (Fig. 11B)

There was a small wound in the second web space and the third toe was warm, red, and swollen.

Footwear and Offloading Aids in Diabetic Foot

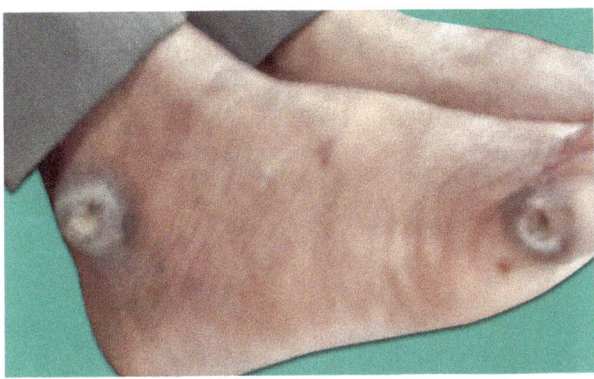

FIG. 10: Callosities over the lateral malleoli and fifth metatarsal head.

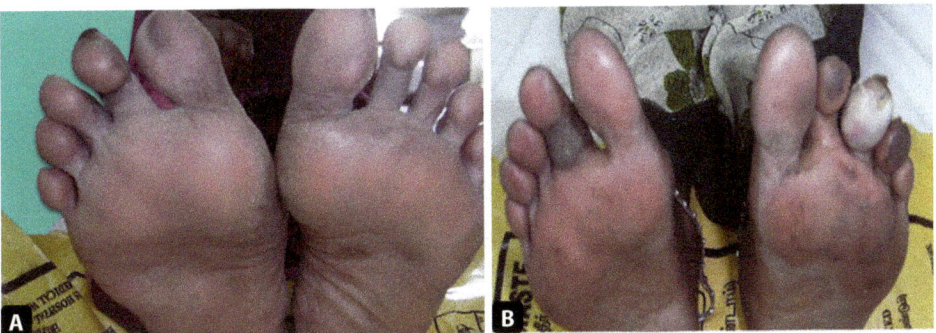

FIGS. 11A AND B: (A) Bilateral toe rings; (B) Swelling and induration in left third toe, callosity in the right second toe.

Intervention

She was prescribed antibiotics, daily cleaning and dressing of the interdigital space, and limited mobility. Strict adherence to not wear toe rings was advised. She was prescribed MCR footwear for indoor as well as outdoor use.

Case 12

A 60-year-old man, known to have T2DM for the last 17 years, presented to the integrated diabetic foot clinic with complaints of a non-healing ulcer over the lateral aspect of the left ankle and deformity for 1 year. History of left little toe ray amputation secondary to gangrene in 2015 and right big toe amputation in 2017.

On Examination (Figs. 12A and B)

Trophic ulcer in the left foot below the lateral malleolus measuring (2 × 3) cm with 1 cm depth exposing the deeper tissues with surrounding callosities was noted. There was a diffuse swelling surrounding the ulcer, which was non-fluctuant, soft, no warmth,

Footwear and Offloading Aids in Diabetic Foot

and non-tender. Also noted to have hyperpigmentation surrounding the ulcer, over the dorsum of the foot and up to the upper one-third of the leg and varus deformity of the left ankle with limb length discrepancy. His X-ray of left foot and ankle showed extensive destruction of the distal ends of tibia, fibula, and tarsal bones (**Fig. 12C**).

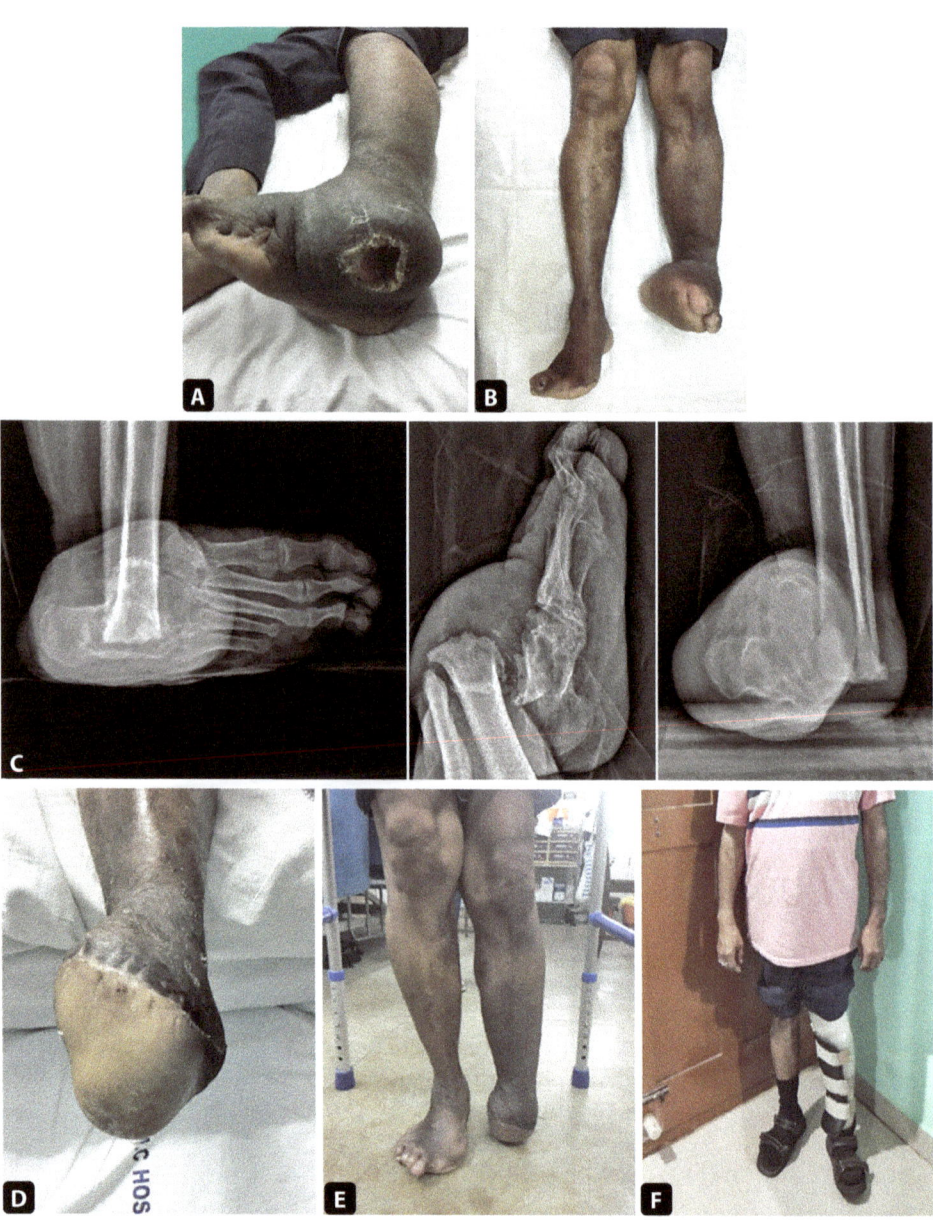

FIGS. 12A TO F: (A) Chronic ulcer over the lateral malleolus of the left foot; (B) Varus deformity of the left ankle with limb length discrepancy; (C) X-ray of the left foot and ankle—anteroposterior and lateral showing extensive destruction of the distal ends of tibia, fibula, and tarsal bones; (D and E) Residual limb post-Syme amputation; (F) With prosthesis.

Intervention

He underwent a left Symes amputation, following which prosthetic training was initiated. He was given a Symes prosthesis once the residual limb was ready.

Syme amputation is disarticulation at the tibiotalar joint with resection of the malleoli. The heel pad is used to cover the end of the tibia. This is an end weight-bearing; ensuring that the patient can weight bear/stand on the limb without use of a prosthesis (**Figs. 12D** to **F**).

CONCLUSION

Foot ulcers are a common complication in persons with DM. This complication frequently leads to lower limb amputation unless a prompt, rational, and multidisciplinary approach to treatment is taken. The main aspects of management that ensures successful and rapid healing of DFU include education, blood sugar control, wound debridement, dressing, offloading, surgery and advanced therapies. When feasible, these approaches should be used to reduce the risk of serious complications such as loss of limb, resulting from foot ulcers. Adaptations of the existing technology to suit the needs of the patient and further research for detecting change in plantar pressures with subtle change in the architecture of the foot and gait is the way forward in management of the patients with diabetes and foot ulcer.

REFERENCES

1. Yazdanpanah L, Nasiri M, Adarvishi S. Literature review on the management of diabetic foot ulcer. World J Diabetes. 2015;6(1):37-53.
2. Martins-Mendes D, Monteiro-Soares M, Boyko EJ, Ribeiro M, Barata P, Lima J, et al. The independent contribution of diabetic foot ulcer on lower extremity amputation and mortality risk. J Diabetes Complications. 2014;28(5):632-8.
3. Dubsky M, Jirkovska A, Bem R, Fejfarová V, Skibová J, Schaper NC, et al. Risk factors for recurrence of diabetic foot ulcers: prospective follow-up analysis in the Eurodiale subgroup. Int Wound J. 2013;10(5):555-61.
4. Schaper NC, Van Netten JJ, Apelqvist J, Lipsky BA, Bakker K; International Working Group on the Diabetic Foot. Prevention and management of foot problems in diabetes: A Summary Guidance for Daily Practice 2015, based on the IWGDF Guidance Documents. Diabetes Metab Res Rev. 2016;32(Suppl. 1):7-15.

CHAPTER 9

ELLIOTT P JOSLIN

Elliot Proctor Joslin (1869–1962) was the first American physician to specialize in diabetes and the founder of the Joslin Diabetes Center. In the 1920s, a 55-year old Joslin took the reins as a global spokesman for the "cause of diabetes." He was the first to advocate for teaching self-care for diabetes to patients, an approach now commonly called DSME (Diabetes Self-management Education). He is also a recognized pioneer in glucose management, identifying that tight glucose control leads to fewer and less severe complications. 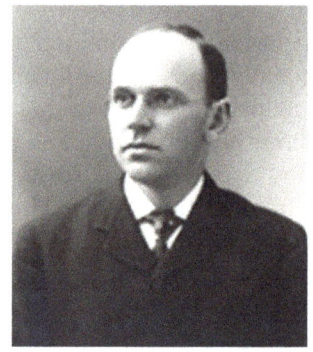 He also advocated foot care for diabetes, setting up a "beauty parlor for feet" staffed with nurses who were instructed to teach the patient to "keep their feet as clean as their face". He also believed that it was "common sense to provide a general hospital for specialization in diabetic surgery". He later recruited McKittrick for the surgical management of diabetes-related lower-extremity lesions.

Callus Removal, Debridement and Foot Care

Bharathi K, Flory Christina I, Ruth Volena D, Shirly Jennifer N, Ezhilarasi V, Sunitha R, Ilakkiya J, Vennela Devarapalli, Felix Jebasingh K, Nihal Thomas

INTRODUCTION

Amongst patients with diabetes mellitus, the prevalence of diabetic foot ulcers (DFUs) has been reported to be 4–10%, with a one-in-four risk of ulceration during an individual's lifetime. Of all amputations associated with a foot wound of any type, DFUs precede up to 83% of major and 96% of minor amputations. Furthermore, it has been reported that 55% of individuals with diabetes and a lower extremity amputation will require further amputation in <3 years. The frequency of mortality of diabetes and diabetes-related complications is greater than the 5-year mortality rate of breast, colon and prostate cancer combined.

Diabetes is a complex disease and the management of DFUs requires input from a wide range of clinical specialties. A multidisciplinary team (MDT) approach to DFUs is key to understanding the linear relationship between uncontrolled diabetes, vascular compromise, foot deformity, diabetic foot infection and other comorbidities. The burden of care and spectrum of services required for sustainable success in diabetic foot care require a team of organized and unified specialist. A team effort along with a systemic approach toward controlling ischemia, wound severity, and foot infection will help reduce the risk of amputation and identify the ever-changing dominant risk factors during a lifetime of the patient's care. Physician, surgeon, vascular surgeon, physical medicine and rehabilitation (PMR) physician, orthotist and prosthetist, physiotherapist and diabetic foot care nurses are required to treat the patient and family.

One of the common findings in the foot is a callous (**Fig. 1**), which is a preceding finding before an amputation.

Callus Removal, Debridement and Foot Care

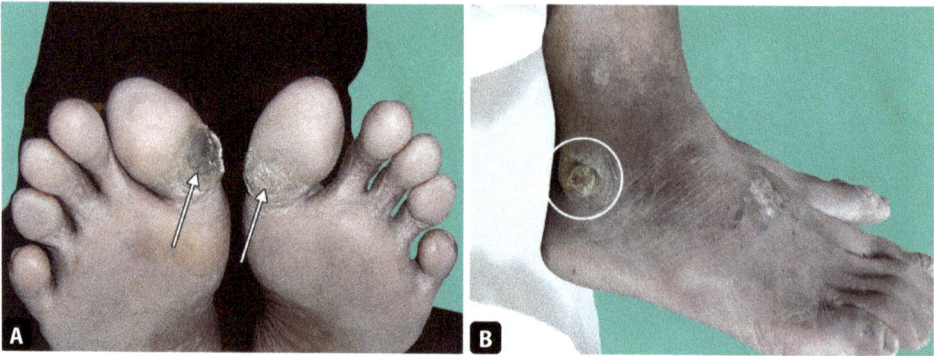

FIGS. 1A AND B: Callous bilaterally in the great toes (shown with the arrows) and over the lateral malleolus (shown with a circle) due to the cross-legged sitting posture.

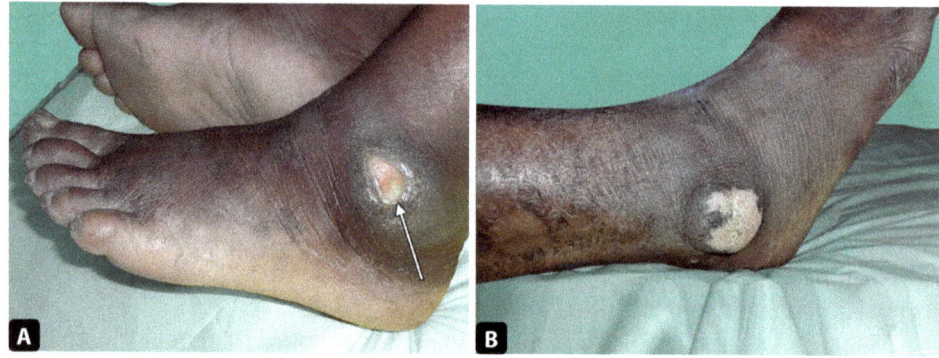

FIGS. 2A AND B: Untreated callous without proper patient education, regarding the cross-legged posture has evolved into a foot ulcer with a healed ulcer over the lateral malleolus in the opposite foot (shown with the arrows).

CALLOUS

- A callosity involves hard skin (hyperkeratosis) (**Figs. 1** and **2**)
- Common sites for callus formation are over bony prominences and in areas subjected to friction, shear and high pressure (often from unsuitable shoes).
- Abnormal anatomy such as hammer toe, claw toe or other deformities such as bunion (due to hallux valgus) can lead to callus formation in the dorsal aspect of the foot (**Figs. 3A** to **F**).
- A callosity in the neuropathic foot is hard and dry due to lack of sweating.[1]

WHY DOES THE CALLOSITY NEED TO BE REMOVED?

- A callosity is a very common precursor of neuropathic ulceration.[2]
- Specks of blood beneath the callosities indicate a preulcerative state (**Fig. 4**).

Callus Removal, Debridement and Foot Care

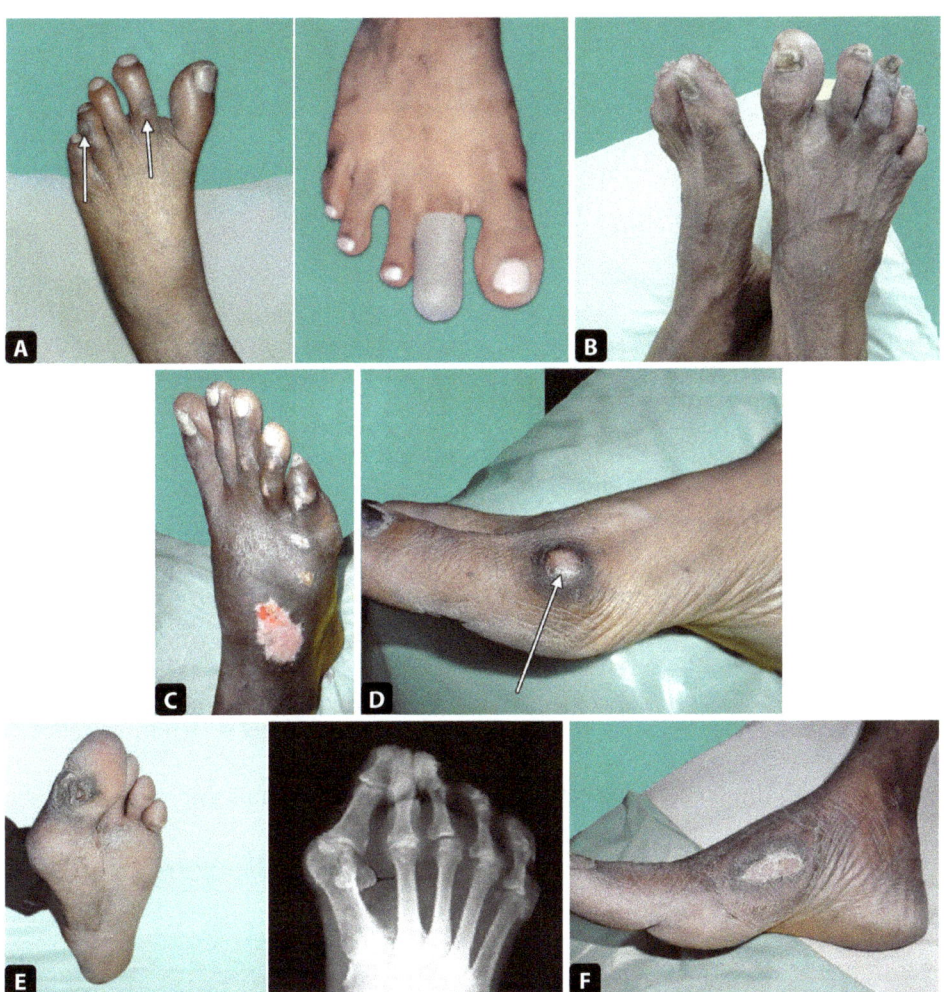

FIGS. 3A TO F: (A) Patient with callosity on the dorsal aspect of the second toe and a foot ulcer in the dorsum of fourth toe, due to friction from the slipper (shown with the arrows) due to clawing of the toes. She was advised a toe cap and a microcellular rubber (MCR) footwear with an anterior rocker; (B) Bilateral claw toes that require a toe cap for the prevention of the foot ulcer on the dorsal and the ventral aspect of the toes; (C) Patient with multiple dorsal foot ulcers due to mild clawing related to the friction from the slippers. She was advised surgical shoes with an anterior rocker with a strap medication to prevent friction with the straps on the footwear; (D) A callosity due to an early bunion on the medial aspect of the great toe (shown with an arrow). He was advised to go for MCR footwear with strap modification so that it prevents friction on the region of the bunion thereby preventing a future ulcer; (E) Bunion with a foot ulcer on the great toe that needs a bunion shield and MCR footwear with an anterior rocker; (F) A callosity with a healed ulcer on the medial aspect of the right foot due to tight commercially available slippers. The patient was advised to wear MCR footwear with a heel counter for better grip and for preventing slippage of footwear due to underlying motor neuropathy.

Callus Removal, Debridement and Foot Care

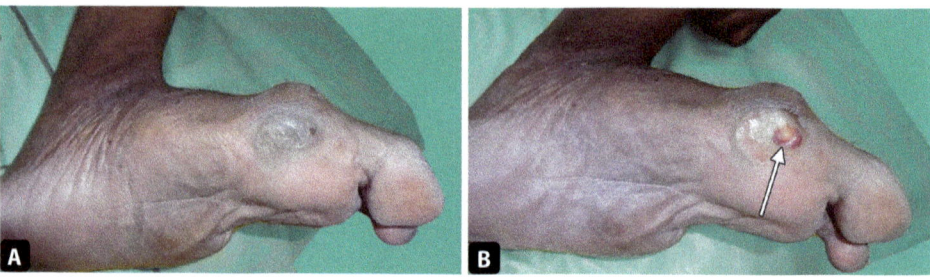

FIGS. 4A AND B: A small hematoma seen after removing the callous (shown with an arrow). The patient was advised to wear microcellular rubber footwear with a strap modification and a 15-degree anterior rocker as he also had clawing of the toes with a previous 4th and 5th toe amputation (not shown in the photographs).

HOW SHOULD CALLUS BE REMOVED?

- The best way to remove a callosity from a high-risk diabetic foot is by sharp debridement (paring with a scalpel by an expert) but should be used with caution in a patient with an ischemic foot).
- Callosities may sometimes be carefully rubbed with a pumice stone by a trained family member.
- Before removing the callus, the skin has to be cleaned either with normal saline or sterile water.
- Place the thumb above the callus area, so that there is stable grip while removing the callus.
- Remove the callus area by debriding it layer by layer, until you feel the normal skin (**Figs. 5A** and **B**).

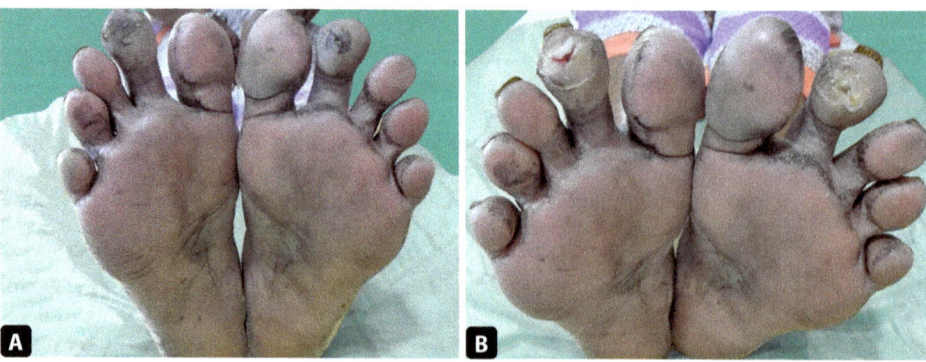

FIGS. 5A AND B: Patient was advised bilateral microcellular rubber footwear with an anterior rocker of 15° to prevent further episodes of callosities.

Callus Removal, Debridement and Foot Care

- A minimal amount of bleeding also indicates the soft layer of the skin (**Figs. 6A** and **B**).
- Callosities are frequently seen around neuropathic ulcers.
- Callosities may grow over an ulcer and prevent exudate from being discharged.
- This frequently leads to infection and further tissue damage.
- Ulcers are slow to heal unless callosities are removed (**Figs. 7** and **8**).

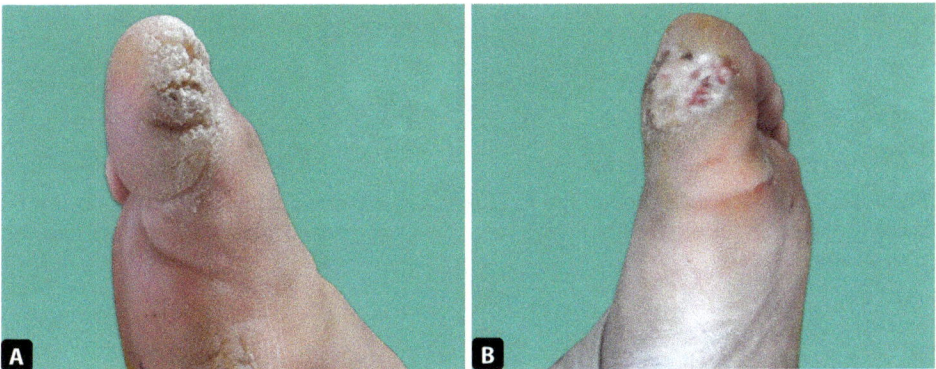

FIGS. 6A AND B: An ulcer at the medial aspect of the right great toe after removal of the callosity. The patient was advised to wear a microcellular rubber footwear with a strap modification. This signifies the importance of debriding thick callous with fissures if not in the weight-bearing areas.

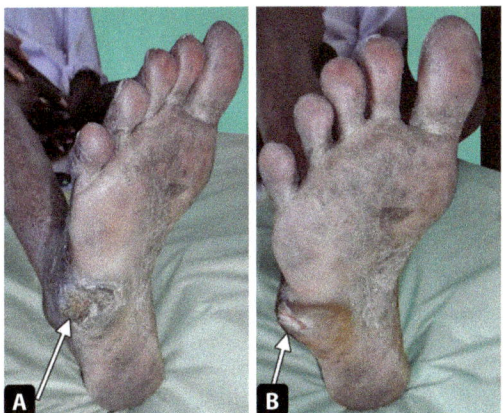

FIGS. 7A AND B: Ulcer detected at the lateral aspect of the left mid foot after the removal of the callosity (shown with the arrows). The patient was advised to use surgical shoes with extra-padding of sponge in the ulcer area.

Callus Removal, Debridement and Foot Care

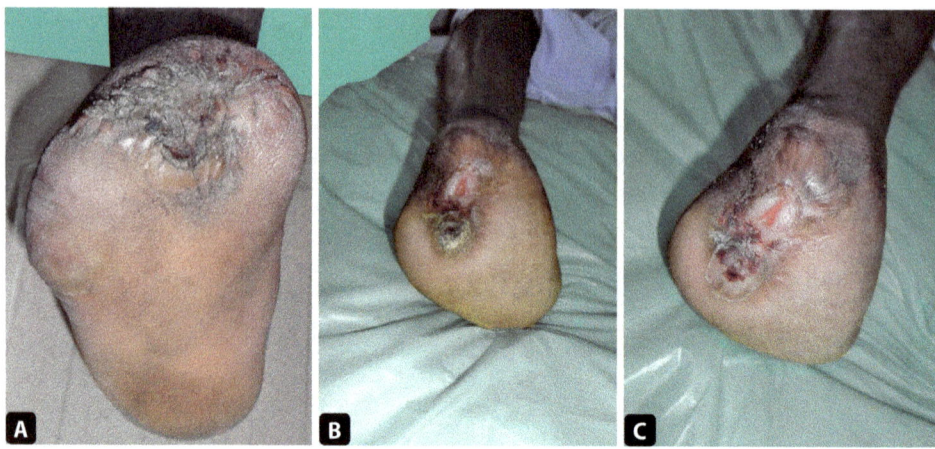

FIGS. 8A TO C: A callosity around the foot ulcer can impair would healing. On removing the callosity, there is an ulcer at the base and the patient was advised to wear customized footwear with an anterior rocker.

FISSURES IN DIABETIC FOOT (FIGS. 9 TO 13)

Fissures in the foot are a common cause for the development of foot ulcers among patients with diabetes mellitus. They commonly develop at the heel.

The pathogenesis of foot ulcers, is in part related to autonomic neuropathy resulting in reduced secretion of sweat thereby leading to fissures. The fissures may extend into the deeper layer, which pose a higher risk of ulceration due to damaged skin. Hence, it is important to treat as well as prevent fissures in the feet in these patients.

Using antikeratotic agents such as salicylic acid, may help in the treatment of fissures. Also, moisturizers such as biolin jelly prevent dryness of the skin.[3]

The initial two patients (**Figs. 10A** and **B**) were given MCR footwear with an anterior rocker and a daily saline dressing. The last two patients (**Figs. 10C** and **D**) were given MCR footwear with a heel counter along with daily dressing.

Common Habits that can Precipitate a Foot Ulcer

Walking barefoot inside as well as outside the house is a major risk factor for the development of foot ulcer. This is due to the fact that these patients do not have decreased or absent sensation in the foot due to the long-standing uncontrolled hyperglycemia. So, all patients should be educated about using footwear all through the day (**Figs. 14A** and **B**).

Wearing tight toe rings or footwear with a toe ring can cause a non-healing ulcer leading on to a local infection and later gangrene that ends with an amputation (**Figs. 15** to **17**). Hence, educating patients on using a footwear with a backstrap, especially in those with motor neuropathy, prevents development of an ulcer.

Callus Removal, Debridement and Foot Care

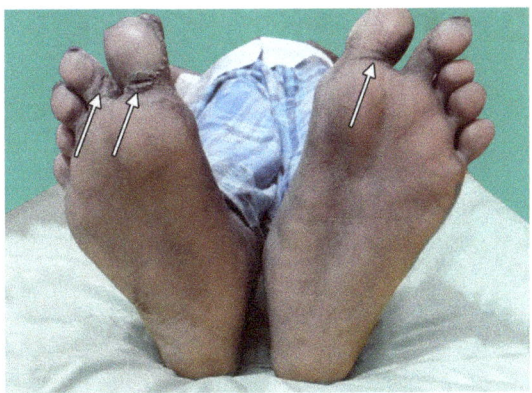

FIG. 9: Fissures at the base of both of great toes and on the right second toe (shown with the arrows). The patient was advised to use microcellular rubber footwear with a 20° anterior rocker and was prescribed 6% salicylic acid for the fissures.

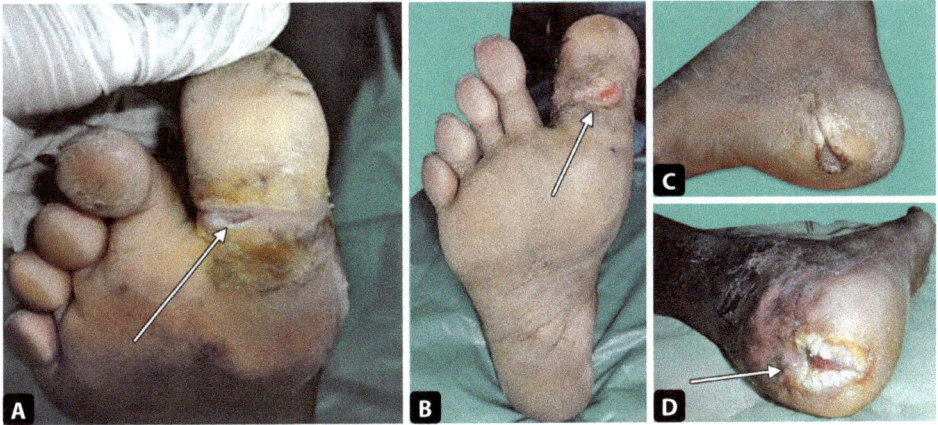

FIGS. 10A TO D: A patient with untreated fissure that had evolved into a foot ulcer (shown with an arrow).

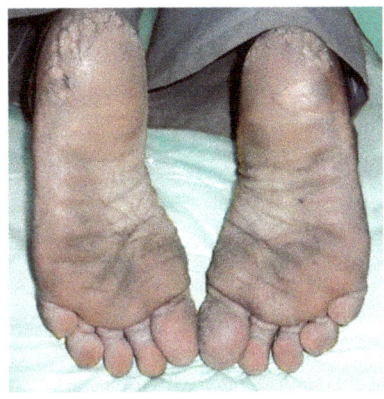

FIG. 11: Fissures over the bilateral hind foot that need urgent care with 6% salicylic acid and appropriate footwear with a heel counter.

Callus Removal, Debridement and Foot Care

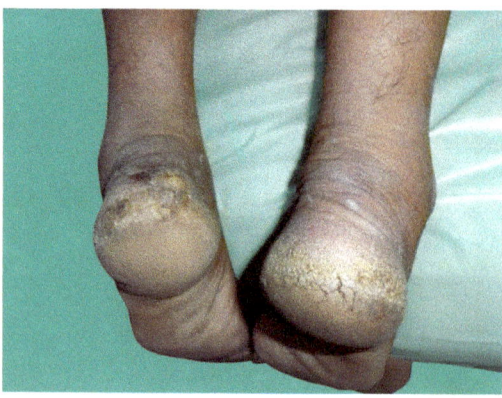

FIG. 12: A fissure on the right foot and a healed ulcer on the contralateral foot due to an untreated fissure. The patient was advised to use microcellular rubber footwear with a heel counter.

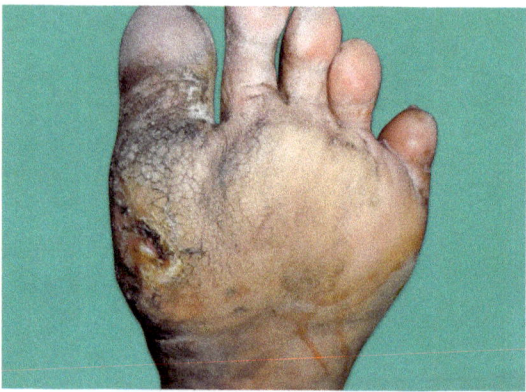

FIG. 13: A fissure with an ulcer that has occurred due to a fissure. The patient was advised to wear microcellular rubber with an anterior rocker and to use 6% salicylic acid for the fissures.

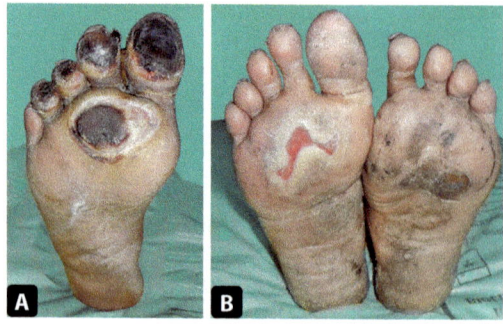

FIGS. 14A AND B: An ulcer that had developed following barefoot walking in the temple. The patient was advised to wear temple socks when going to temple. For long-term use, he was advised to wear microcellular rubber footwear with an anterior rocker as he had a previous left great toe amputation.

Callus Removal, Debridement and Foot Care

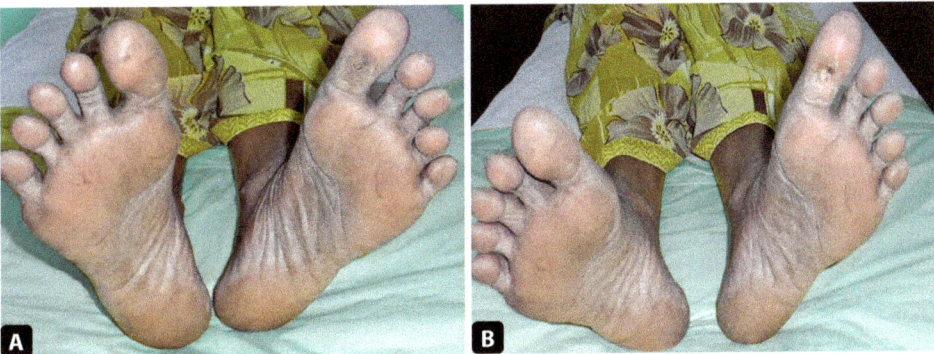

FIGS. 15A AND B: Use of toe rings can be detrimental in patients with diabetes and neuropathy. This patient has a callosity in the great toe. After scraping the callosity, there is a small ulcer at the base. She was advised to wear microcellular rubber footwear with an anterior rocker thereafter.

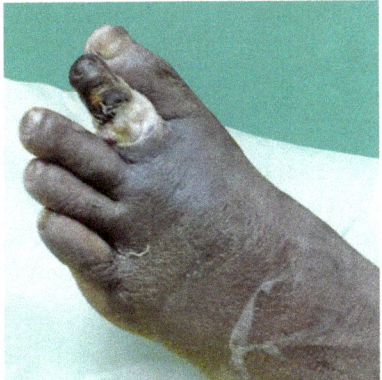

FIG. 16: A tight toe ring causing an ulcer and gangrene of the left second toe. The patient required an amputation of the toe.

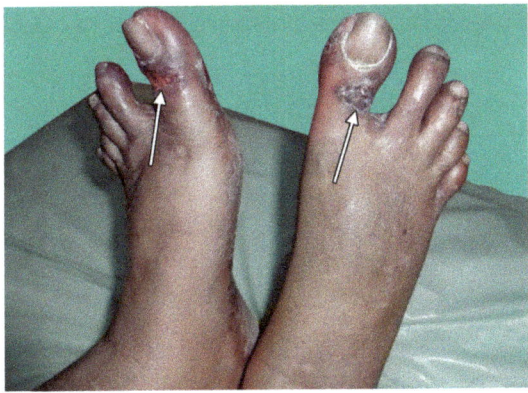

FIG. 17: Bilateral great toe dorsal foot ulcers due to commercially available footwear with a toe ring (shown with the arrows). The patient was advised microcellular rubber footwear with an anterior rocker.

Callus Removal, Debridement and Foot Care

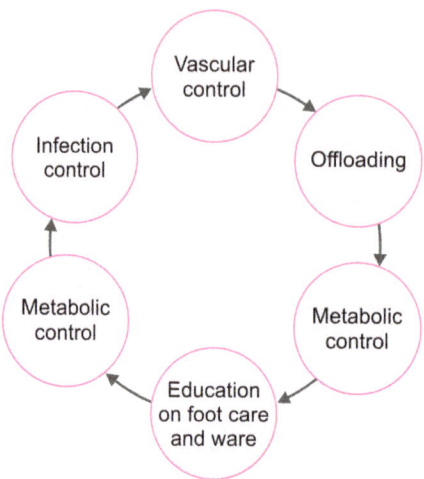

FIG. 18: A Multi-disciplinary approach toward diabetic foot therapy.

Managing the Diabetic Foot

The management of foot ulcers requires a multidisciplinary approach. With simple modifications of footwear, one can avoid foot ulcers in future, particularly in those patients with severe neuropathy. Moreover, patients should be educated to inspect the foot and the footwear to prevent development of new foot ulcers (**Fig. 18**).

REFERENCES

1. Arosi I, Hiner G, Rajbhandari S. Pathogenesis and treatment of callus in the diabetic foot. Curr Diabetes Rev. 2016;12(3):179-83.
2. Pataky Z, Golay A, Faravel L, Da Silva J, Makoundou V, Peter-Riesch B, et al. The impact of callosities on the magnitude and duration of plantar pressure in patients with diabetes mellitus. A callus may cause 18,600 kilograms of excess plantar pressure per day. Diabetes Metab. 2002;28(5):356-61.
3. Oe M, Sanada H, Nagase T, Minematsu T, Ohashi Y, Kadono T, et al. Factors associated with deep foot fissures in diabetic patients: a cross-sectional observational study. Int J Nurs Stud. 2012;49(6):739-46.

Callus Removal, Debridement and Foot Care

FOOT CARE: INFORMATION FOR PATIENTS

Foot Examination

- Examine the feet daily with the help of mirror (**Fig. 1A**) to look for dry skin (**Fig. 1B**), callus, fissures (**Fig. 1C**), new-onset redness, any color changes, blister and skin breakdown.
- Advise the patient not to forget to check in between the toes for fungal infestation (**Figs. 1D** and **E**) and the back of the heels.
- To instruct to inspect after any trauma, no matter how minor, to the feet.

Soak and Scrub (Figs. 2A to C)

- Wash the feet in lukewarm water and dry them carefully in between the toes.
- For dry skin or cracks, soak the feet in lukewarm water for 15–20 minutes and then scrub with the help of nylon scrubber or pumice stone.
- Use a moisturizer every day (but not between your toes) for dry skin and cracking.

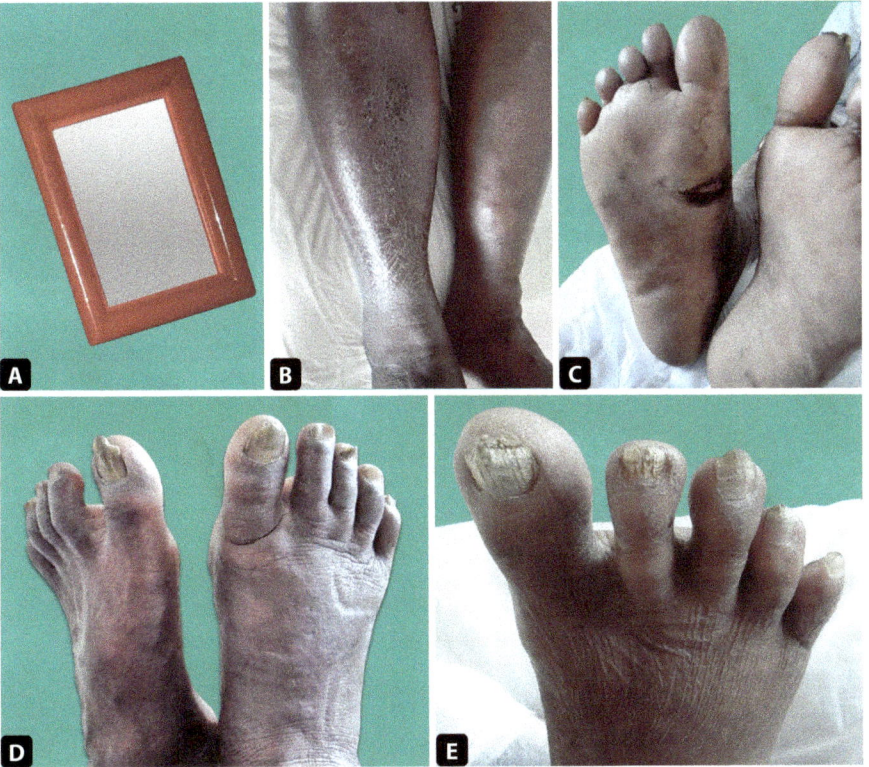

FIGS. 1A TO E: (A) Mirror to look at the plantar aspect of the foot; (B) Dry skin over the shin of the tibia; (C) Fissures; (D and E) Fungal nail.

Callus Removal, Debridement and Foot Care

Nail Care

- Always cut nails with safety clipper, never with scissors.
- Cut them straight across and leave plenty of room out from the nailbed.
- After cutting the nails, nicely file the edges gently with nail file.
- If client has problem with vision or using hands, get help from a family member.
- A family member needs to be trained to do nail trimming in a safe manner (**Fig. 3**).

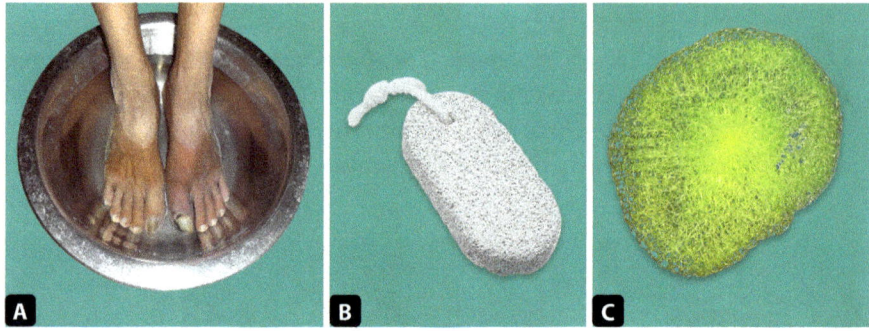

FIGS. 2A TO C: (A) Soak and scrub in the warm water; (B) Pumice stones; (C) Scrubber.

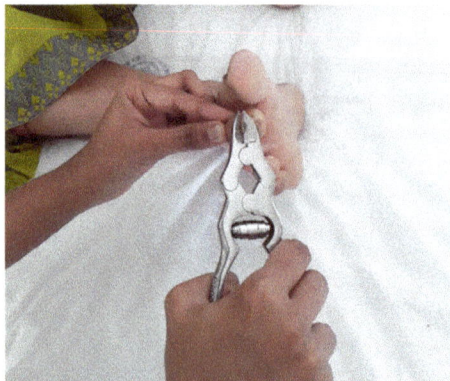

FIG. 3: Trimming of thickened nail with a bone cutter.

Callus Removal, Debridement and Foot Care

Suitable Shoes

- Unsuitable shoes or shoes that do not fit properly are the most common cause of foot problems with diabetes.
- Check the feet every time while removing shoes. Also remember to remove socks, stockings or tights and check for any redness or blisters.
- Check the bottom of the shoes before putting them on to make sure that nothing sharp such as a pin, nail or glass has pierced the outer sole.
- Also, run the hand inside each shoe to check and ensure that no small objects such as small stones are hidden inside.
- Wear well-fitting shoes. Make sure the shoes are long enough, deep enough, and wide enough for the feet.
- If shoes are too tight, they will compress the toes.
- When buying new shoes, always try on both shoes simultaneously. Wear new shoes around the house for short periods (20 minutes) and then check the feet.
- Look for problems such as redness caused by rubbing or pressure.

Do's

- Inspect your feet daily
- Wash your feet in lukewarm water
- Be gentle when cleaning your feet
- Moisture your feet
- Cut nails straight and file corners
- Check shoes and feel inside before wearing
- Keep feet warm and clean
- Take care of your diabetes
- Use microcellular rubber footwear for diabetes

Don'ts

- Never treat corns or callus yourself
- Do not wash your feet in hot water
- Avoid wearing tight socks
- Avoid moisture in between the toes
- Do not cut nails in the corners
- Do not use adhesive tapes on your feet
- Do not keep feet dry
- Do not smoke
- Never walk barefoot

Callus Removal, Debridement and Foot Care

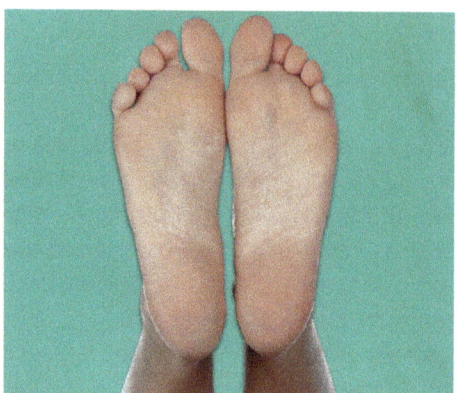

"Think of the magic of that foot, comparatively small, upon which your whole weight rests. It's a miracle, and the dance…is a celebration of that miracle."

— **Martha Washington**

CHAPTER 10

FREDERICK TREVES

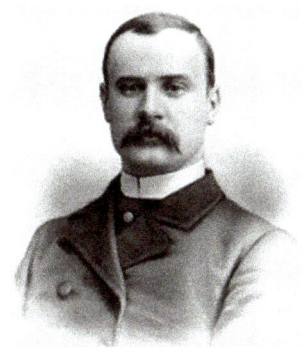

Toward the end of the 19th century, another important contribution to diabetic foot care was made by Frederick Treves. He suggested an alternative approach for the treatment of ulcers, using sharp debridement of callus after application of linseed poultices to soften the callus. After debridement, he applied an antiseptic to the thin, fresh epidermis. Once the patient was mobilized, he instructed the patient to wear a thick pad of felt plaster over the healed ulcer. This was done to reduce pressure and prevent recurrence of the wound. Therefore, by doing this, Treves had established three important principles in the treatment of ulceration of the foot: (i) sharp debridement, (ii) off-loading pressure, and (iii) education about foot care and appropriate footwear.

Negative Pressure Wound Therapy

Ida Nirmal, Albert Abhinay Kota, Bharathi K, Felix Jebasingh K

CASE SCENARIO

A 68-year-old lady, diagnosed to have long-standing type 2 diabetes mellitus and peripheral neuropathy presented to the integrated diabetes foot clinic with a history of a non-healing ulcer of the dorsal aspect of the right foot of 1-year duration. She received multiple courses of oral and intravenous (IV) antibiotics and underwent debridement multiple times in the past. On examination, she had an (11 × 5) cm ulcer on the dorsal aspect of the right foot with poor granulation tissue and no signs of infection. X-ray of the right foot did not show evidence of osteomyelitis.

She underwent extensive debridement to remove necrotic tissue and slough to the maximum extent possible. After debridement, a foam-based dressing was done over the wound under aseptic precautions. The dressing was covered with adhesive tape to create an airtight seal. An evacuation tube embedded in foam was connected to a fluid collection canister contained within a portable vacuum machine. Negative pressure was applied intermittently thrice a day. Negative pressure wound therapy (NPWT) dressing was changed as and when required. Healthy granulation tissue started appearing during the first week of therapy and complete wound healing occurred by 6 weeks after the initiation of therapy.

Negative pressure wound therapy also referred to as topical negative pressure therapy is a useful treatment for a variety of acute and chronic wounds and, unlike many other wound treatments and dressings, has a relatively sound evidence base to demonstrate its effectiveness. Complex wounds may benefit from negative pressure therapy. Consideration may be given to the appropriate patient selection and dressing application.

Total negative pressure (TNP) technology, which is informally referred to as "wound vac," is also known by several other pseudonyms, including the following:
- Vacuum-assisted closure (VAC)
- Vacuum-sealing technique (VST)
- Sealed surface wound suction (SSS)
- NPWT

The five key points of NPWT are as follows:
1. NPWT has been found to help in healing many complex wounds.
2. This therapy can be used in both acute and chronic settings.
3. Practitioners using NPWT must be trained to use the specific device.
4. The patient selection must involve assessing a range of factors in addition to the wound requiring treatment.
5. It must be applied carefully to avoid damaging the wound bed or causing pressure damage to the surrounding skin.

Indications for using NPWT include the following:
- *Acute wounds*: Trauma, amputation, burns, abdominal wounds, and sternotomy wounds
- *Chronic wounds*: Pressure sores, failed skin grafts, diabetic foot ulcers, and venous/stasis ulcers

Contraindications for NPWT include the following:
- Wounds involving untreated osteomyelitis
- Wounds exposing blood vessels or vascular grafts or organs or with an unexplored fistula
- Wounds including open joint capsules
- Skin malignancy and excised skin malignancy—except for palliative care
- Wounds with necrotic tissue

Relative contraindications for NPWT are as follows:
- Wounds with a visible fistula
- Coagulation disorder (risk of bleeding)
- Compromised microvascular blood flow to the wound

Patient selection for NPWT is as follows:
Patients whose wounds are suitable for NPWT need to be assessed for their ability to live with the device. The following factors should be considered:
- Level of mobility and risk of tripping: Drain tubes can create a trip hazard for those with reduced mobility, who may also find the larger pumps too cumbersome.
- The level of cognitive ability and risk of pulling the dressing or tubes off
- Mental health status and ability and willingness to adhere to the treatment regimen, which involves always wearing the pump and having two or three dressing changes a week, and to care for the pump.
- The position of wounds or wounds and the ability to obtain and maintain a seal
- Pain at dressing changes—some patients may need a pain killer for pain relief

MECHANISM OF ACTION

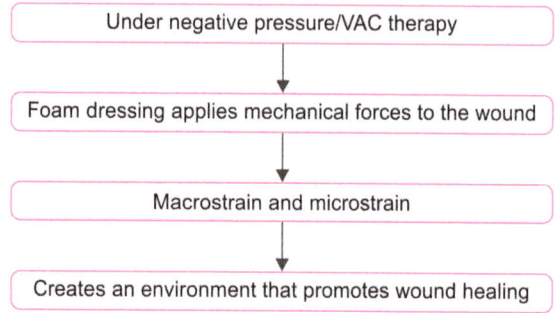

Macrostrain

It is the visible stretch that occurs when negative pressure contracts the foam that:
- Draws wound edges together
- Provides direct and complete wound bed contact
- Positive pressure to the wound surface (5–10 mm Hg)
- Removes exudate and infectious materials

Microstrain

Microstrain is the microdeformation at the cellular level, which leads to cell stretch thereby:
- Reduces edema
- Promotes perfusion
- Promotes granulation tissue formation by facilitating cell migration and proliferation.

The treatment is thought to assist healing by providing a moist environment and removing interstitial fluid and exudate; and enhancing granulation tissue formation, angiogenesis, and tissue perfusion. Others have reported fluctuations in blood flow, which may be useful in patients with compromised vascularity.[1-3]

Equipment Needed for Negative Pressure Wound Therapy
- VAC machine and canister
- VAC foam and drape
- Non-collapsible evacuation tube
- Sterile scissors and gloves
- Wound cleansing pack
- Normal saline
- Adhesive tape

STEPS OF APPLYING NEGATIVE PRESSURE WOUND THERAPY

- Wash hands.
- Prepare the dressing articles.
- Open the wound.
- Prepare the wound.
- Place the foam dressing on the wound.
- Place an air vent.
- Apply the drape (transparent film-Opsite™) over the dressing.
- Secure the dressing, connect the noncollapsible tube to the suction catheter.
- Connect the suction catheter to the canister of the wall suction (continuous suction).
- Record the dressing procedure with information like the condition of the wound, size, and depth of the wound, dressing material used, pressure adjustment (mm Hg), and condition of the patient.

TECHNIQUE OF THE PROCEDURE

- The foam dressing is cut to the approximate size of the wound with scissors (**Fig. 1**).
- Foam is placed gently into position (**Fig. 2**).
- The perforated drain tube is then located on top of the foam and the second piece of foam is placed over the top (**Fig. 3**).
- For a shallow wound, a single piece of foam may be used, and the drainage tube is
- inserted inside it.
- Foam and surrounding few inches of the healthy skin is covered with a transparent film (**Fig. 4**).

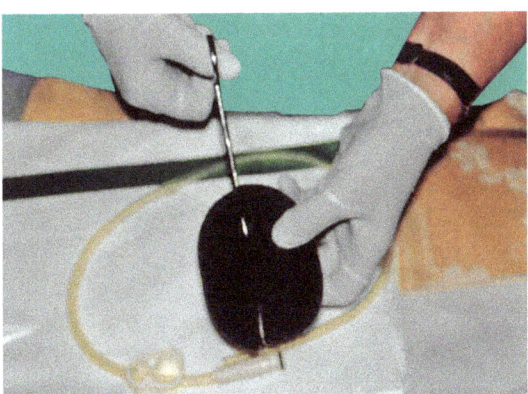

FIG. 1: The foam dressing is cut to the approximate size of the wound with scissors.

Negative Pressure Wound Therapy

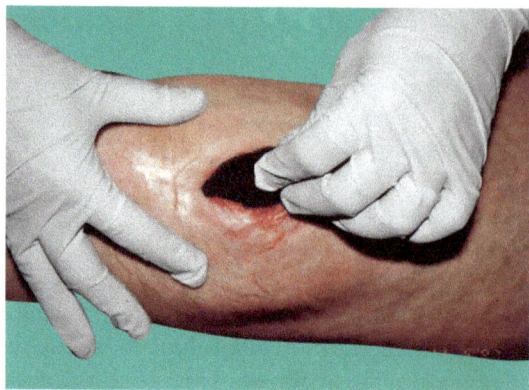

FIG. 2: Foam is placed gently into position.

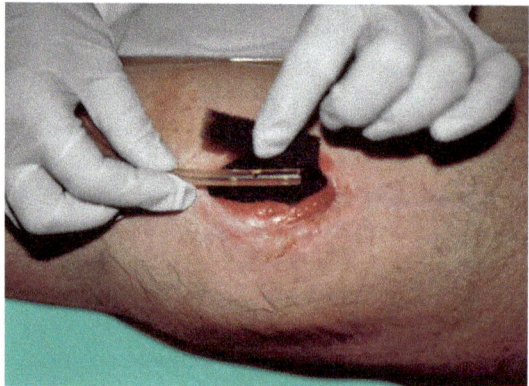

FIG. 3: The perforated drain tube is then located on top of the foam and the second piece of foam is placed over the top.

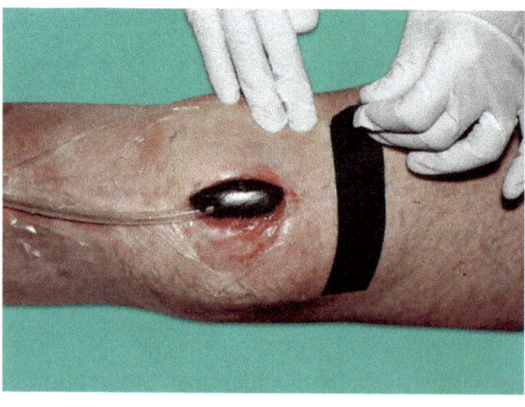

FIG. 4: Foam and surrounding few inches of the healthy skin are covered with a transparent film.

Negative Pressure Wound Therapy

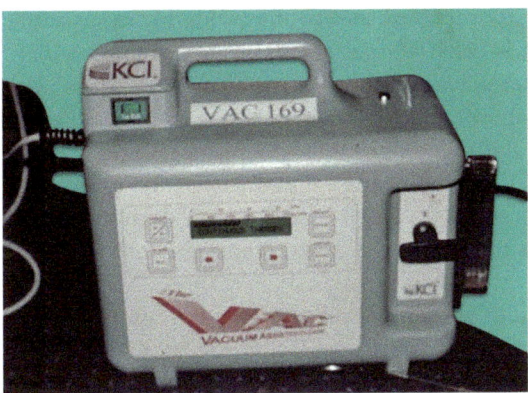

FIG. 5: The distal end of the drain is connected to the vacuum-assisted closure (VAC) unit, which is programmed to produce the required level of pressure.

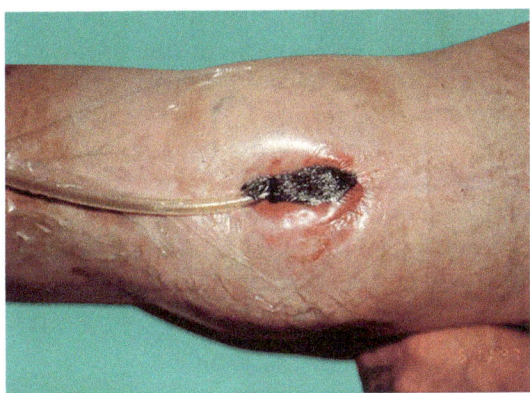

FIG. 6: Once the vacuum is switched on, the air is sucked out of the foam causing it to collapse inward drawing the edges of the wound in with it.

- The distal end of the drain is connected to the VAC unit, which is programmed to produce the required level of pressure (**Fig. 5**).
- Once the vacuum is switched on, the air is sucked out of the foam causing it to collapse inward drawing the edges of the wound in with it (**Fig. 6**).

Practitioners applying NPWT must ensure that:
- Healthy skin is not damaged by contact with foam, gauze, or drains. Exposed tissues such as tendon or bone are not damaged.
- Dressing materials are not left to embed into granulation tissue.
- Drains do not cause pressure damage.
- Patients and staff are familiar with the functionality of the pump.

- Foam/gauze does not come into contact with the intact skin.
- The intact skin is lined with a film dressing if foam needs to extend onto it, for example with small wounds or when bridging more than one wound.
- When more than one piece of foam or gauze is used, no gaps are left between the pieces.
- An airtight seal is created using a film dressing.
- For drains secured on top of the dressing, if the drain port is larger than the wound, it must not extend beyond the dressing margin onto the skin, to prevent pressure damage.

The application of NPWT dressings is not difficult but it requires an understanding of how the therapy works and training in the use of the specific device. Staff undertaking dressing changes should have the appropriate knowledge and training—poor dressing technique can lead to wound complications or breaches in the seal. The wound is filled with gauze or foam, depending on the device used, then a drain is applied to facilitate the application of negative pressure and remove wound exudate.

Drains are either inserted into the wound filler or on top, again depending on the device. Any areas of undermining, tracks, or sinuses must be fully explored and filled to ensure negative pressure is achieved at these deepest areas. Carving foam is a skilled procedure as it involves creating a shape that fits into the wound contours. If more than one piece of foam is used, it is important to document how many so they can be counted out at dressing change. The wound bed should be thoroughly examined for flecks of foam or threads of gauze at dressing change so that these can be removed. It is also necessary to secure drains at the exit point of the dressing to help obtain a seal and to prevent skin damage due to pressure at the exit point.

The benefits of NPWT are as follows:
- Enhanced healing and granulation tissue formation
- Management of highly exuding wounds
- Reduced dressing changes compared with more conventional dressings
- Reduced nurse time
- Reduced costs
- Improved quality of life

Complications of NPWT include the following:
- Pressure necrosis from the tubing
- The trauma of periwound skin
- Growth of granulation tissue into foam
- Allergic reaction to the drape
- Fistula formation
- Neoplasm caused by an increase in blood flow and rate of healing

WHEN SHOULD VACUUM-ASSISTED CLOSURE BE DISCONTINUED?

- Psychological intolerance/non-concordance with VAC therapy
- No healing response within 1 week of commencing VAC therapy
- Frank pus in the dressing or canister
- Uncontrolled/excessive bleeding or hematoma under the dressing

EVIDENCE OF NEGATIVE PRESSURE WOUND THERAPY IN DIABETIC FOOT ULCERS

Negative pressure wound therapy aids in the management of diabetic foot ulcers by the physical and biological effects that influence the healing of these ulcers. NPWT causes numerous alterations in the wound environment that include removal of excess exudate, stimulation of senescent cells, mobilization of macrophages, and stimulation of angiogenesis.

Armstrong et al. published a randomized controlled trial (RCT) that demonstrated the benefit of NPWT compared to standard care in the time to heal and the proportion of wounds healed in 162 patients with postoperative diabetic foot wounds.[4] Blume et al. in their RCT comparing NPWT to moist wound therapy using hydrogels and alginates in diabetic foot ulcers found that 43% of the wounds healed completely in NPWT healed at 16 weeks compared to 29% in the moist therapy ($p = 0.007$) and a smaller number of minor digit amputations in the NPWT group. In a Cochrane review of 44 RCTs and five economic studies by Gill et al., surgical wounds treated prophylactically with NPWT experienced fewer surgical site infection (SSI) compared to standard dressings and NPWT had varied cost-effectiveness (**Fig. 7**).[5-10]

The cost of adding NPWT may be significant if this modality is applied to the outpatient setting, and hence this form of advanced wound care is better utilized in in-hospital stay and for large, complex wounds.

To summarize, NPWT is an alternative/adjunctive wound care therapy for complex traumatic, infective or dehisced postoperative wounds and diabetic foot ulcers.

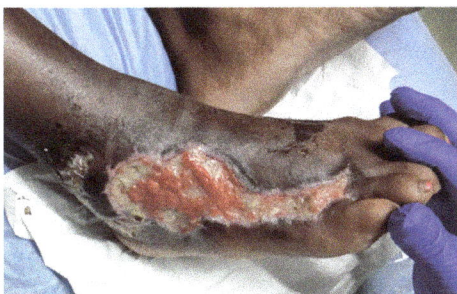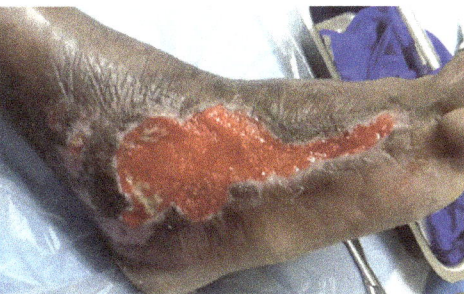

FIG. 7: Before and after 1 week of negative pressure wound therapy (NPWT).

REFERENCES

1. Norman G, Goh EL, Dumville JC, Chiverton L, Scuffham P, Stankiewicz M, et al. Negative pressure wound therapy for surgical wounds healing by primary closure. Cochrane Database Syst Rev. 2020;3(3):CD009261.
2. Peinemann F, Labeit A. Negative pressure wound therapy: A systematic review of randomized controlled trials from 2000 to 2017. J Evid-Based Med. 2019;12(2):125-32.
3. Älgå A, Haweizy R, Bashaireh K, Wong S, Lundgren KC, von Schreeb J, et al. Negative pressure wound therapy versus standard treatment in patients with acute conflict-related extremity wounds: a pragmatic, multisite, randomised controlled trial. Lancet Glob Health. 2020;8(3):e423-9.
4. Armstrong DG, Lavery LA, Diabetic Foot Study Consortium. Negative pressure wound therapy after partial diabetic foot amputation: a multicentre, randomised controlled trial. Lancet Lond Engl. 2005;366(9498):1704-10.
5. Berger P, de Bie D, Moll FL, de Borst G-J. Negative pressure wound therapy on exposed prosthetic vascular grafts in the groin. J Vasc Surg. 2012;56(3):714-20.
6. UpToDate. Negative pressure wound therapy. [online] Available from: https://www.uptodate.com/contents/negative-pressure-wound-therapy?search=negative%20pressure%20wound%20 therapy&source=search_result&selectedTitle=1~68&usage_type=default&display_rank=1. [Last accessed November. 2021].
7. Huang C, Leavitt T, Bayer LR, Orgill DP. Effect of negative pressure wound therapy on wound healing. Curr Probl Surg. 2014;51(7):301-31.
8. Vikatmaa P, Juutilainen V, Kuukasjärvi P, Malmivaara A. Negative Pressure Wound Therapy: a Systematic Review on Effectiveness and Safety. Eur J Vasc Endovasc Surg. 2008;36(4):438-48.
9. Zens Y, Barth M, Bucher HC, Dreck K, Felsch M, Groß W, et al. Negative pressure wound therapy in patients with wounds healing by secondary intention: a systematic review and meta-analysis of randomised controlled trials. Syst Rev. 2020;9(1):238.
10. Ichioka S, Watanabe H, Sekiya N, Shibata M, Nakatsuka T. A technique to visualize wound bed microcirculation and the acute effect of negative pressure. Wound Repair Regen Off Publ Wound Heal Soc Eur Tissue Repair Soc. 2008;16(3):460-5.

LELAND McKITTRICK

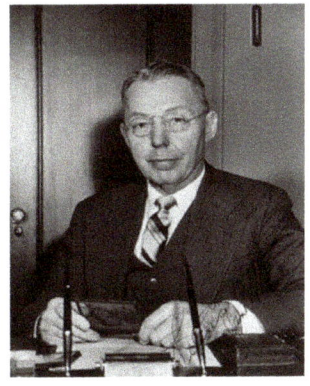

Leland McKittrick, MD (1893–1978) was recruited by Dr Elliot P Joslin to provide for the surgical management of lower-extremity lesions in patients with diabetes at the New England Deaconess Hospital. His contributions to the field were wide-ranging. He recognized that the amputation of the great toe, with its metatarsal head, had altering effects on weight-bearing, increasing the susceptibility of the foot (toes and metatarsals) to further injury. Thus, he preferred the "relative security" and safety of the transmetatarsal amputation. Dr McKittrick was later joined by the general surgeon Frank C Wheelock Jr, MD who became interested in the emerging field of vascular surgery. He was the first American surgeon to use an end-to-side femoral popliteal bypass graft. Drs McKittrick, Wheelock, Carl Hoar, and John Rowbotham established an unparalleled reputation of the New England Deaconess Hospital, for the management of the surgical complications of diabetes, including minor amputations and distal bypasses.

Surgery of the Diabetic Foot

Pranay Gaikwad

INTRODUCTION

It is better to understand the foot afflictions in diabetes mellitus as a constellation of syndromes that may broadly be considered as diabetic foot disease (DFD). The three most important components of DFD are— (i) diabetic foot ulcer (DFU), (ii) diabetic foot infection (DFI), and (iii) diabetic foot osteomyelitis (DFO). Foot infections (inframalleolar) contribute a significant threat to the limb and life of a person with diabetes. With increasing the incidence of diabetes, DFIs are responsible for increasing a common cause for hospitalization, amputations, and deaths. Analogous to the cancer survival statistics, the estimated 5-year survival in DFI is <50%.

The onset of DFD often begins with DFU. Often arising as a result of poorly controlled diabetes, other factors discussed in the previous sections may contribute as well. As the spectrum of presentation varies, the management can range from simple conservative measures upto major amputations.[1] This chapter will deal with the surgical management of DFU presuming that the patient is receiving medical treatment concurrently.

EPIDEMIOLOGY

It is estimated that nearly a third of persons with diabetes have the lifetime risk of developing DFU and half of these individuals will develop DFI in some form (**Box 1**).

BOX 1: Common types of diabetic foot infection (DFI).	
• Paronychia	• Necrotizing soft tissue infection*
• Cellulitis	• Septic arthritis
• Abscess	• Osteomyelitis
*Includes infection of subcutaneous fat, fascia, and muscles.	

The risk factors for DFI include:
- Open wound
- Chronic ulcer
- Previous amputation
- Peripheral arterial disease
- Peripheral neuropathy
- Renal failure
- Ill-fitting footwear/walking barefoot

PATHOGENESIS

Neuropathy is central in the causation of a DFU and its progression to the DFI. Simply put, motor neuropathy affects the muscles of the foot changing to new areas of weight bearing. Sensory neuropathy further alters the foot mechanics causing osteoarticular and osteoarthropathy with the development of callus and skin ulceration. Dryness of the skin because of autonomic neuropathy leads to fissures and spontaneous skin breakdown. The coexistence of the peripheral arterial disease leads to tissue hypoxia and impaired migration of leukocytes to the site of infection. With the impairment of leukocyte and monocyte function, compromised immune defenses further contribute to the onset and perpetuation of infection in DFU.[2]

SURGICAL MANAGEMENT

Surgical management of DFD can be either preventive or therapeutic but often the treatment is also preventive for future complications. In acute settings, therapeutic intentions prevail over preventive interventions, while the converse is true for chronic wounds.

SURGICAL MANAGEMENT WITH THERAPEUTIC INTENT

Removal of all infection and necrotic tissues remains the basic tenet of surgical management of DFD. The problem is often underestimated until the patient presents in an acute setting. Therefore, a systematic approach is recommended (**Box 2**).

On a wider scale, surgical treatment is often remembered as the three 'D's viz. decompression, drainage, and debridement. To this, a fourth 'D' in the form of drug therapy may be added.

BOX 2: Stepped approach in the surgical treatment of diabetic foot infection (DFI).

- Incision at the infection site
- Inspection of tissues in the depths of infection
- Debridement of devitalized tissues
- Culture from the wound: Soft tissue and bone
- Irrigation
- Hemostasis
- Postoperative care

Decompression begins with a "layered" incision and drainage of tissues until the tissue involved deepest is reached. Debridement is the removal of foreign matter and necrotic tissue from a wound. Excision of necrotic tissues including the involved tendons and bone is done; a decision that is based on clinical, radiological, and intraoperative findings. Bone is resected one joint above the level of bone infection.

Surgical Debridement

Active foot infections with ulcers necessitate surgical intervention according to the severity of the infection. The urgency and magnitude of the procedure is determined by the clinical condition and the extent of involvement. Only infections limited to the superficial tissues such as cellulitis or lymphangitis may be managed by non-operative means. Common indications and options for an urgent surgical intervention are listed in **Boxes 3** and **4**.

Most DFUs, that are not life-threatening/limb-threatening, are initially treated with surgical debridement. Additionally, minor debridement may be done using chemical or enzymatic agents. The extent of debridement may vary, but it provides an opportunity to examine the site of entry of the infection and obtain a specimen for culture. Moreover, surgical debridement of DFU allows examining the wound, especially evaluation of the deeper tissue planes even up to the underlying bone or joint.

Due to sensory neuropathy and inability to visually appreciate the ulcer in its initial stage, the infection progressively spreads to and destroys the deeper tissues until it reaches a point when it manifests as a full-blown infected DFU with a spectrum of necrotizing infection. Consequently, the timing of surgical intervention determines its magnitude, the length of stay in the hospital, and the outcome. The extent of surgical procedures can range from debridement, fasciotomy to minor or major amputations. Removal of all devitalized tissue and drainage of collections remains the basic tenet in the treatment of any DFU. In all but the most critically sick patients, efforts should be directed toward as complete a debridement as possible in the first instance itself, to avoid the need for further debridement. Despite the best initial efforts, due to further proximal extension of the infection and worsening sepsis, multiple procedures may be required in some patients (**Box 2**).

BOX 3: Indications for surgical interventions in diabetic foot ulcer (DFU).

- Necrotizing fasciitis
- Extensive necrosis
- Gangrene
- Crepitus or gas in tissues (on imaging)
- Critical ischemia
- Life-threatening sepsis

BOX 4: Surgical options for diabetic foot ulcer (DFU).

- Fasciotomy
- Debridement
- Amputation: minor/major

The magnitude of surgical treatment is inversely proportional to the preservation of the limb and its functionality. After initial sepsis is treated with thorough debridement of devitalized tissues, every effort must be made to minimize the loss of non-devitalized tissue and preserve its primary function, weight bearing and ambulation. Likewise, post-procedure deformities leading to altered foot dynamics should be avoided. A clear understanding of the vascularity of the limb with DFU is a must for revascularization and early rehabilitation. In some situations, the infection and tissue destruction have gone far enough that it may threaten the patient's life when a major amputation is the only alternative. Despite best efforts, a minority of patients will succumb to the severity of sepsis and comorbidities.[3]

Antibiotic Therapy

At presentation, infection in DFU should be categorized as per the PEDIS (Perfusion Extent Depth Infection Sensation) grade. Antibiotic therapy is indicated in the presence of active infection. The features of active infection in DFU can vary from swelling, induration, redness, pain, warmth, and discharge. Once the grade of infection is established, its treatment may be planned appropriately. Similarly, the continuation of antibiotics, beyond a limited course that was sufficient to eradicate infection, has not been required to accomplish the healing of ulcers that remain open (**Table 1**).

During the management of DFI, features of DFO should be looked for as it has bearing on the outcome of the treatment. Clinical features need to be correlated with laboratory and radiography findings (**Box 5**).

TABLE 1: Infection in diabetic foot ulcer (DFU) (as per PEDIS* Grade).

Grade of infection	Antibiotic therapy
Grade 1: No infection	Not required
Grade 2: Infection involving skin and subcutaneous tissue	Broad-spectrum based on likely organisms
Grade 3: Infection involving deeper tissues but no SIRS	Broad-spectrum before wound management
Grade 4: Any foot infection with SIRS	Broad-spectrum along with wound management

*Perfusion Extent Depth Infection Sensation.
(SIRS: systemic inflammatory response syndrome)

BOX 5: Features favoring diabetic foot osteomyelitis (DFO).

- Ulcer larger than 2 cm^2
- Extends up to bone (wound probe test)
- ESR >70 mm/h
- Raised serum CRP
- Imaging:
  - Plain radiograph—foreign bodies, soft tissue gas, osteolytic changes, periosteal elevation
  - Magnetic resonance imaging

Antibiotic Therapy for Diabetic Foot Infection

In most situations, a culture specimen is obtained from the wound and broad-spectrum antibiotic therapy is initiated. Subsequently, with the availability of the sensitivity patterns, a more directed approach should be adopted. This is best decided as per the local hospital infection control committee (HICC), but a general approach may be as follows:

- *Acute, mild, or moderate infection*: Commonly due to gram-positive organisms such a *Staphylococcus* and *Streptococcus* may be treated with cephalexin or amoxicillin-clavulanate.
- *Specific organisms* may be treated with an appropriate antibiotic (methicillin-resistant *Staphylococcus aureus* (MRSA), pseudomonas, etc.).
- *Superficial DFU* with extensive cellulitis may be treated with antibiotics that cover *Streptococcus* and *Staphylococcus*.
- *Necrotic wounds* with a fetid odor may need anaerobic microbial coverage
- *Severe infections with systemic inflammation* often need the most advanced broad-spectrum antibiotics such as carbapenems, β-lactamase inhibitors, teicoplanin, or vancomycin (carbapenem therapy is associated with fewer failures). Currently, there is no high-level evidence to support the use of topical antimicrobial agents in the management of DFI. Newer delivery systems such as biodegradable vehicles (calcium sulfate beads impregnated with antibiotics) and natural polymers (collagen sponge) are emerging as promising prospects.

The duration of antibiotic treatment depends upon the time course of the clinical response, which is generally 1–2 weeks. After the acute infection is under control, the regimen may be converted to appropriate orally bioavailable antibiotics. The need for adequate debridement cannot be over-emphasized in limiting the required duration of antibiotic therapy. Antibiotic therapy is reviewed with the availability of culture results and clinical response, usually after 3–5 days of commencement. Sometimes, the current therapy may be continued in the cases with a satisfactory clinical response despite resistant bacteria, except in cases with MRSA, where specific agents must be used. Conversely, with an unsatisfactory clinical response in the presence of bacterial resistance, it is prudent to assess the wound for deep-seated abscess or necrosis as well as vascular insufficiency. The antibiotics can be discontinued once the infection has resolved, even if the ulcer is yet to heal completely. Persistent non-infected DFUs should be managed with wound care and non-weight bearing to eliminate the portal of entry of infection. Extended antibiotic therapy is required to treat *Staphylococcal* sepsis which may be associated with seeding of other sites such as cardiac valves, bones, and joints.

Antibiotic Treatment of Diabetic Foot Osteomyelitis

The treatment of DFO is much debated. The argument rages between minimal debridement with a long course of antibiotics to aggressive debridement with excision of all infected bone. Selection of treatment strategy should be individualized based on several factors (**Table 2**).

TABLE 2: Roles of medical therapy and surgical therapy.

Primarily medical therapy with minimal debridement	Aggressive debridement
To avoid foot dysfunction due to surgery	Failure of medical therapy
Limb ischemia	Life-threatening infection
Excessive risk of surgery	Extensive bone necrosis
Osteomyelitis limited to forefoot with minimal soft tissue infection	Foot remodeling for function
Patient preference	Antibiotic toxicity
	Patient preference

TABLE 3: Duration of antibiotics in diabetic foot osteomyelitis (DFO).

Extent of debridement	Antibiotics as per	Duration of antibiotics
Infected bone completely removed	Soft tissue culture	2–3 weeks
Limited or no bone debridement	Bone culture	6 weeks or more

Optimal antibiotic therapy of DFO involves the treatment of both soft tissue infection and bone infection; antibiotic therapy should be based on precise microbial cultures and sensitivity (**Table 3**).

Despite best efforts, infection may persist and a protocol should be designed to review the patient and the wound at regular intervals. Causes of persistence of infection can be:
- Inadequate vascularity
- Persistent soft tissue or bone necrosis in the depths
- Inadequate cover for specific organisms (e.g., MRSA)
- Antibiotic resistance
- Ineffective antibiotic bioavailability
- Improper nonweight bearing
- Non-compliance to treatment

As per the findings, the treatment should be modified appropriately.

Adjunctive Therapy

Besides surgical treatment and antibiotic therapy, the management of DFD should optimally involve a multipronged approach. These include:
- Wound care:
  - Non-adherent dressings
  - Offloading
  - Revascularization
- Glycemic control
- Reconstructive surgery

Many novel methods for management (hyperbaric oxygen, platelet-derived growth factor, skin equivalents, granulocyte colony-stimulating factor, topical injection of stem cells, negative-pressure wound therapy, etc.) have been tested but not enough evidence exists to support their routine use. Likewise, topical antibiotics have not been proven to be better than standard wound treatment while they may also result in adverse reactions or antibiotic resistance.

SURGICAL PREVENTIVE STRATEGIES

These include both non-surgical and surgical methods. Some of the non-surgical methods that have been alluded to earlier, include a good glycemic control, attention to foot hygiene, well-fitting footwear and offloading through a total contact cast. Surgical intervention is directed toward the restoration of blood supply, redistribution of pressure points and prevention of life-threatening sepsis (**Table 4**).

Amputation as a Preventive Strategy

Despite ordinarily being the last resort in the management of DFI/DFO, amputations do play an important role in planning rehabilitation and expediting a chronic non-healing wound with a non-functional or dysfunctional foot limiting the patient's mobility. Proper rehabilitation of an affected limb may be protective for the contralateral "precious" limb. However, it is not uncommon in diabetics when sequentially both lower limbs may get affected. While the urgency of amputation may be dictated by the presence of systemic inflammation, the level of amputation is decided as per the involvement of the bone or joint and vascularity of the foot/limb. Amputations are generally considered as partial when limited to foot and high-level when done above the ankle[4] (**Table 5** and **Fig. 1**).

OUTCOME

With appropriate care, a satisfactory clinical response can be anticipated in 90% of patients with mild non-limb-threatening infection and at least 60–80% of those with moderate or severe limb-threatening infection. Limb-threatening infections may require foot-sparing amputations, but the salvage of a weight-bearing foot is

TABLE 4: Interventions in preventive strategies.

Preventive strategy	Surgical procedure
Revascularization	Angioplasty +/− stenting and bypass graft
Podiatric procedures	Achilles tenotomy and exostectomy of Charcot neuroarthropathy
Plantar flexion deformity correction	Hammer and Mallet toe correction
Arthrodesis	Severe mid- or hindfoot Charcot deformity
Life-threatening sepsis	Amputation at appropriate level

TABLE 5: Types and levels of amputations in diabetic foot osteomyelitis (DFO).

Type of amputation	Skeletal level
Partial amputation	Toe amputation
	Ray amputation: Single or multiple
	Transmetatarsal amputation
	Tarsometatarsal amputation (Lisfranc)*
	Transverse tarsal amputation (Chopart)*
	Calcaneal partial resection and fusion to tibia (Pirogoff)*
	Distal trans tibiofibular amputation (Syme)*
High-level	Below knee amputation
	Above-knee amputation

*Uncommon.

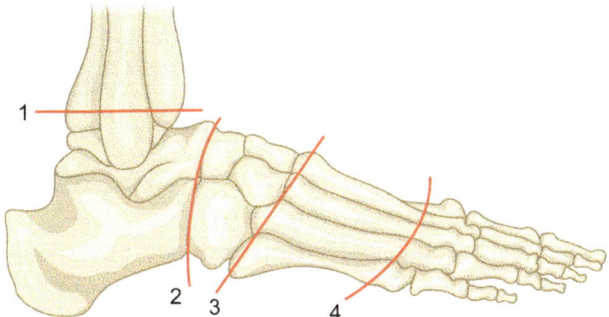

FIG. 1: Levels of foot amputations: (1) Syme, (2) Chopart, (3) Lisfranc, and (4) Transmetatarsal.

usually achievable. Vascular reconstruction, especially bypass grafts to pedal arteries which restore pulsatile flow to the foot, decrease major amputations and enable foot-sparing/foot-salvage surgery. Although the clinical science of treating DFIs has advanced significantly, challenges remain in defining optimal care. Even so many foot infections can be prevented, effective therapy provided and extremities salvaged if current knowledge is more widely applied.

REFERENCES

1. Frykberg RG, Wukich DK, Kavarthapu V, Zgonis T, Dalla Paola L. Board of the Association of Diabetic Foot Surgeons. Surgery for the diabetic foot: A key component of care. Diabetes Metab Res Rev. 2020;36 Suppl 1:e3251.
2. Piaggesi A, Apelqvist J (eds). The Diabetic Foot Syndrome. Front Diabetes. Basel, Karger. 2018;26:184-99.
3. Setacci C, Sirignano P, Mazzitelli G, Setacci F, Messina G, Galzerano G, de Donato G. Diabetic foot: surgical approach in emergency. Int J Vasc Med. 2013;2013:296169.
4. Weledji EP, Fokam P. Treatment of the diabetic foot - to amputate or not? BMC Surg. 2014;14:83.

CHAPTER 12

ALFRED-JEAN FOURNIER

Alfred-Jean Fournier was born in Paris on May 12, 1832, into a family with a medical background. He attended and excelled at the Institution Jauffret, at the Lycee Charlemagne, and the Concours General. He is famous for his propositions on the origins of syphilis, which he believed was a cause of the symptoms of symptoms of paralysis, motor incoordination, and progressive locomotor ataxia. His contribution to necrotizing fasciitis was by describing the Fournier's gangrene (a type of necrotizing fasciitis) as a "fulminant gangrene of the penis and scrotum in young men". It is often a rare, but serious complication of diabetes mellitus.

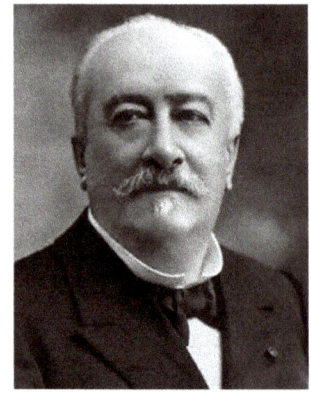

Necrotizing Fasciitis in Diabetes

Pranay Gaikwad

INTRODUCTION

Soft-tissue infections have affected mankind since time immemorial. Necrotizing soft-tissue infections (NSTIs) can involve superficially from the skin right up to the bone. This condition is marked with fulminant tissue destruction (hence the term "flesh-eating") with signs of systemic sepsis and even death. Prompt diagnosis and treatment are critical for reducing morbidity and mortality. The true incidence of NSTIs is difficult to estimate owing to variable and inconsistent reporting.

NSTIs are further subcategorized according to several, sometimes descriptive, schemes. They are classified as per the (1) primary anatomic structure and depth of the infection, (2) anatomic region of the body, (3) type of microorganisms involved in the infection, or (4) presence of gas within the tissues (**Table 1**).

TABLE 1: Classification of necrotizing soft-tissue infections.

Classification	Features
Anatomic location	• Fournier gangrene—perineum/scrotum • Meleney ulcer—abdominal wall
Depth of infection (correlates with mortality)	Necrotizing adipositis (most common), fasciitis, and myositis
Microbial cause	• *Type I*: Polymicrobial (most common, 55–75%) • *Type II*: Monomicrobial (*Staphylococcus, Streptococcus,* and clostridia) • *Type III*: *Vibrio vulnificus* • *Type IV*: Fungal/MRSA
Presence of gas	• Clostridial infections • Non-clostridial infections

(MRSA: methicillin-resistant *Staphylococcus aureus*)

As the necrotizing infection spreads into the deeper tissues, the line of distinction between the diagnosis of necrotizing fasciitis (NF) and necrotizing myositis blurs and other components in the spectrum of NSTIs can coexist in a patient.[1]

NECROTIZING FASCIITIS

This is an infection of the deep fascia with progressive destruction of the superficial and deeper tissues. The deep fascia is vulnerable because of its poor vascularity. Clinically, while the patient may have features of sepsis, the local finding in NF can be quite deceptive in its initial stages. On a cursory examination, the overlying skin may look *and feel* deceptively normal. As the clinician's experience grows, the characteristic tenderness and induration of the underlying tissues become unmistakable. With time, the necrotic infection may progress with the overlying skin developing an area of anesthesia. Further progression is marked with the appearance of blebs, ecchymoses, and cutaneous necrosis. Unfortunately, even at this late stage, the diagnosis can be confirmed only with the inspection of the fascia.

Type I (Polymicrobial) Necrotizing Fasciitis

The infection is caused by both aerobic and anaerobic bacteria. The type of organisms may vary according to the anatomical site involved (**Table 2**).

Diabetes with the associated peripheral arterial disease is the most common predisposing factor for type I NF. Other comorbid factors may contribute to the aggravation or seriousness of the condition (**Box 1**).

TABLE 2: Microbes involved in necrotizing fasciitis.

	Anatomical site	**Organisms**
Type I	All sites	• *Anaerobes*: *Bacteroides*, *Clostridium*, and *Peptostreptococcus* • *Aerobes*: Enterobacteriaceae (*Escherichia coli*, *Enterobacter*, *Klebsiella*, and *Proteus*)
	Fournier gangrene	*Anaerobes*: *Bacteroides*, *Fusobacterium*, *Clostridium*, anaerobic or microaerophilic streptococci
	Head and neck	• *Aerobes*: *E. coli*, *Klebsiella*, and enterococci • *Anaerobes*: *Fusobacteria*, anaerobic streptococci, *Bacteroides*, and Spirochaetes
Type II	Upper aerodigestive tract, trauma, and muscle strain	Group A *Streptococcus* (GAS) and *Staphylococcus*
Type III	• Trauma in freshwater • Trauma in seawater	• *Vibrio vulnificus* • *Aeromonas hydrophila*
Type IV		*Candida* species

BOX 1: Risk factors for necrotizing fasciitis.

- Diabetes
- Peripheral arterial disease
- Trauma
- Recent surgery
- Immunosuppression
- Malignancy
- Obesity
- Alcoholism
- Pregnancy
- Drugs:
  - Sodium-glucose cotransporter-2 inhibitors
  - Nonsteroidal anti-inflammatory drugs

Type II (Monomicrobial) Necrotizing Fasciitis

The NF due to group A *Streptococcus* (GAS) can occur in healthy persons with no comorbidities. Virulence of GAS may be variable and the strains of GAS with the M protein types 1 and 3 can cause toxic shock syndrome (TSS).

CLINICAL FEATURES

In patients with diabetes, the lower extremities are more commonly affected by NF than in other areas. The presentation is either acute or acute-on-subacute infection (**Fig. 1**).

Initially, the subcutaneous tissue feels firm and indurated with the underlying muscles becoming less distinct on palpation. In contradistinction to the cardinal features of acute inflammation, there is a paradoxical loss of sensation in the affected area because of thrombosis of small blood vessels and the destruction of superficial nerves in the subcutaneous tissue. This sign, when present, is suggestive of the diagnosis of NF. The presence of surgical emphysema in the subcutaneous tissues is further contributory evidence of type I NF. Concomitantly, the color of the skin changes from normal to red-purple to blotchy patches of blue-gray. Eventually, the skin breaks down with blebs containing pinkish-purple fluid and gangrene. Severe pain with loss of motor function and disappearance of distal pulses are suggestive of a compartment syndrome.

There is a rapid deterioration over hours resulting in systemic inflammatory response leading to limb loss, organ failure, and death. Consequently, timely recognition and treatment are of paramount importance.[2] Common clinical features are listed in **Table 3**.

INVESTIGATIONS

Laboratory findings are suggestive of a systemic inflammatory response due to the ongoing infective process (**Box 2**).

Despite the derangement in the above mentioned laboratory parameters, the diagnosis of NF cannot be predicted with certainty. A scoring tool like "Laboratory Risk

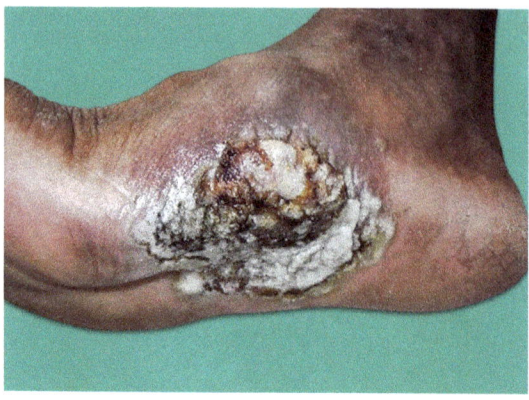

FIG. 1: Acute-on-chronic presentation of necrotizing soft tissue infection.

TABLE 3: Clinical features in necrotizing fasciitis.

Local findings	Systemic manifestations

• Erythema (without sharp margins)
• Edema extending beyond the visible erythema
• Severe pain (out of proportion to exam findings)
• Fever
• Crepitus
• Skin blebs, ecchymosis, or necrosis
	• Symptoms:
	  ○ Malaise
	  ○ Myalgias
	  ○ Diarrhea
	  ○ Anorexia
	• Signs:
	  ○ Fever
	  ○ Tachycardia
	  ○ Hypotension

BOX 2: Laboratory findings in necrotizing fasciitis.

- Leukocytosis with shift to the left
- Metabolic acidosis with hyponatremia
- Coagulopathy
- Raised inflammatory markers (C-reactive protein and/or erythrocyte sedimentation rate)
- Elevated serum creatinine and lactate
- Elevated creatine kinase and aspartate aminotransferase suggest deep infection involving muscle or fascia (as opposed to cellulitis)

Indicator for Necrotizing Fasciitis" (LRINEC) has been shown to aid in the diagnosis but not exclude NF. A recent systematic review and meta-analysis has revealed that a score ≥6 has a sensitivity of 68.2% and specificity of 84.8% for the diagnosis of NSTI. Consequently, LRINEC has not found too many advocates (**Table 4**).

TABLE 4: Laboratory Risk Indicator for Necrotizing Fasciitis (LRINEC) scoring tool.

Variable	Score
C-reactive protein (mg/dL):	
<15	0
≥15	4
White blood cell (WBC) (/mm^{-3}):	
<15,000	0
15,000–25,000	1
≥25,000	2
Hemoglobin (g/dL):	
>13.5	0
11–13.5	1
<11	2
Sodium (mmol/L):	
≥135	0
<135	1
Creatinine (mg/dL):	
≤1.6	0
>1.6	1
Glucose (mg/dL):	
≤180	0
>180	1

Note: Blood culture and sensitivity are useful in guiding antibiotic therapy.

Imaging

In general, the diagnosis is suspected in any patient with the above features and further supported by radiological imaging. However, in the presence of crepitus, surgical intervention should not be delayed. The choice of imaging will depend upon the condition of the patient and the available resources. If the renal function is normal, the contrast-enhanced computed tomography (CT) scan can demonstrate the presence of gas in tissues, fluid collections, and inflammatory changes around the deep fascia. Magnetic resonance imaging (MRI) tends to overestimate the soft tissue inflammation besides being time-consuming in a sick patient. Musculoskeletal ultrasonography can be readily done at the bedside that may provide information on fluid collections, necrosis, and even gas in tissues but is operator dependent. However, no imaging modality can conclusively diagnose NF therefore, the diagnosis can be made only by surgical exploration.

The diagnosis of necrotizing infection is established via surgical exploration of the suspected area in the operating room with the physical examination of the skin, subcutaneous tissue, fascial planes, and muscle with the characteristic macroscopic findings. Due to necrosis, there is a lack of tissue resistance to a probing finger along the fascial planes (finger test) (**Box 3**).

Further, surgical exploration helps evaluate the scope of involvement and to debride devitalized tissue. Importantly, when NF is suspected, surgical exploration should not be delayed while awaiting the laboratory or imaging results. A complete microbial assay should be done for all intraoperative specimens, to subclassify the NF and to decide upon the most appropriate agent(s). This includes the culture and sensitivity for aerobes, anaerobes, and fungus. The histopathology of the tissues is not necessary to make the diagnosis of NF but is recommended (**Box 4**).

TREATMENT

Principles of Treatment

Treatment of necrotizing infection consists of early and aggressive surgical exploration and debridement of necrotic tissue, together with broad-spectrum empiric antibiotic therapy, and hemodynamic support.

Surgical Treatment

The surgical treatment is, in effect, a variable extent of debridement. Survival is best when the surgical intervention is undertaken within 6 hours, while it is significantly poor with the delays over 24 hours (**Table 5**). Antibiotic therapy without surgical intervention has a near 100% mortality rate (**Fig. 2**).

BOX 3: Intraoperative features of necrotizing fasciitis.

- Swollen and dull-gray necrotic tissue
- Lack of bleeding
- Thrombosed vessels
- Thin exudate—"Dishwater" pus
- Noncontractile muscle
- Positive "finger test"

BOX 4: Pathological features of necrotizing fasciitis.

- Extensive tissue destruction
- Thrombosis of blood vessels
- Bacteria along the fascial planes
- Presence of acute inflammatory cells

TABLE 5: Surgical options in necrotizing fasciitis (NF).

Procedure	Indication
• Superficial fasciotomy	Necrosis limited to the skin and subcutaneous fascia
• Deep fasciotomy	NF with impending compartment syndrome
• Amputation:	
○ Minor	• Extensive NF spreading to muscle, across joints
	• Distal soft tissue necrosis with proximally extending NF
○ Major	• Life-threatening NF or extensive soft tissue necrosis[3]

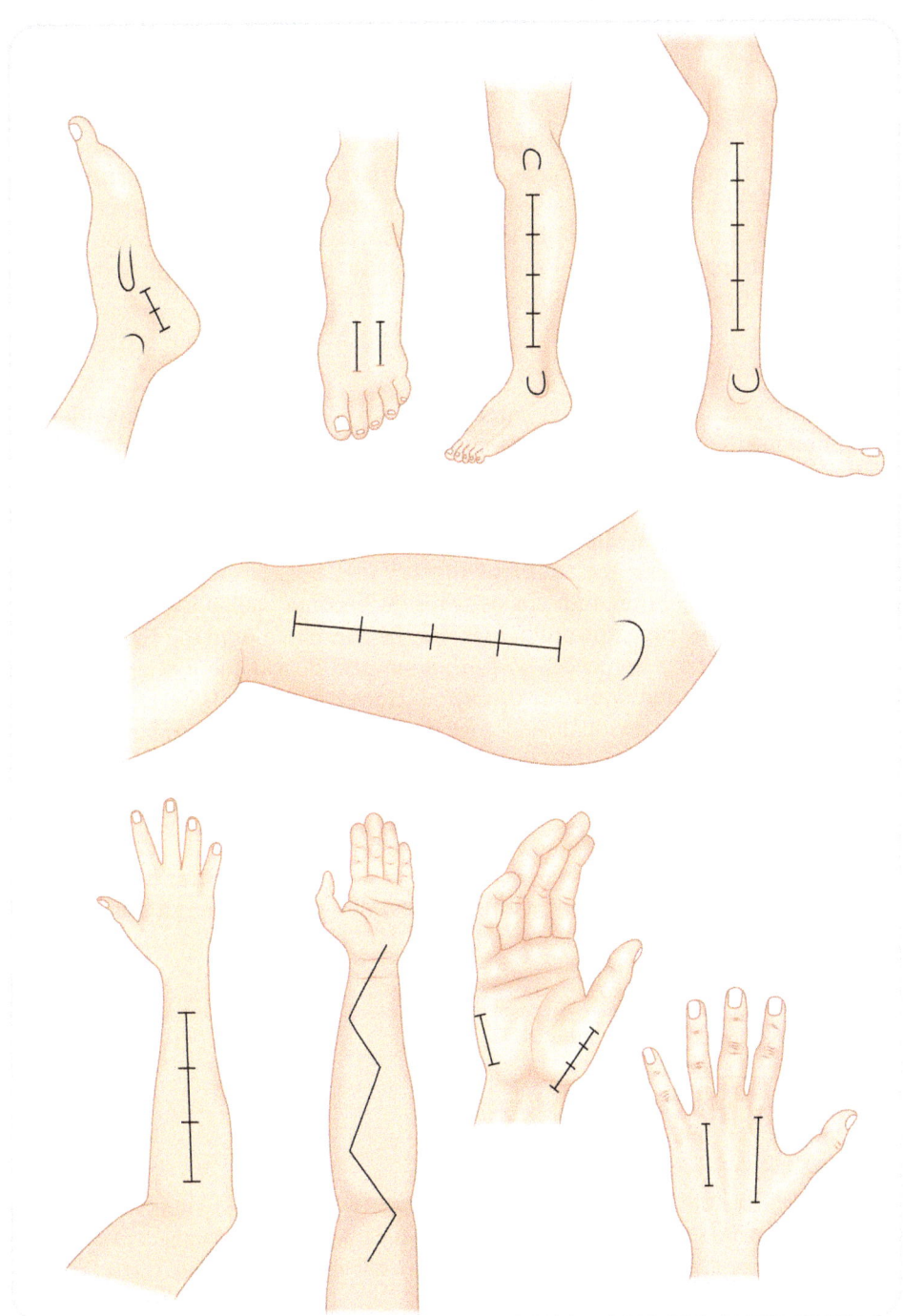

FIG. 2: Fasciotomy incisions for necrotizing soft-tissue infection of extremities.

Surgical Debridement

Necrotizing fasciitis is a surgical emergency. Radiographic imaging studies should not delay surgical intervention when there is crepitus on examination or rapid progression of clinical manifestations.

The goal of operative management is to perform aggressive debridement of all necrotic tissue until healthy, viable (bleeding) tissue is reached. The wound should be inspected every day and continued to be debrided until all the necrotic tissue is removed. Amputation, minor or major, remains the last resort to control the severe necrotizing infection involving the extremities.

Antibiotic Therapy

Necrotizing fasciitis is a serious condition that requires prompt intervention. At presentation, the empiric treatment should begin after obtaining blood cultures with the administration of broad-spectrum antimicrobial therapy that covers against gram-positive, gram-negative, and anaerobic organisms. The type of empiric antibiotic may be based on the local Hospital Infection Control Committee (HICC) recommendations. Later, the antibiotic therapy may be converted to more specific antibiotic(s) as the cultures and sensitivity results become available (**Box 5**).

As a general principle, the antibiotics may be continued until the source-control of the sepsis has been achieved, no further surgical debridement is required, and the hemodynamic condition is near-normal. However, the decision to discontinue antibiotics should be individualized for each patient based on several factors such as renal function, liver function, and resistance.

Hemodynamic Support

Depending upon several factors such as delay in seeking medical treatment, the seriousness of the longstanding comorbid conditions, and the virulence of the

---

BOX 5: Common empiric antibiotic regimens in necrotizing fasciitis.
- Carbapenem group of antibiotics
- Piperacillin-tazobactam
- Additional antibiotics for specific organisms:
    - Vancomycin/daptomycin (MRSA infection)
    - Penicillin (β-hemolytic streptococci)
    - Clindamycin (toxin elaborating strains of streptococci/staphylococci and clostridia)
    - Trimethoprim-sulfamethoxazole/cephalosporins/carbapenems (freshwater *Aeromonads*)
    - Doxycycline + ceftriaxone/cefotaxime (marine-water infection with *Vibrio vulnificus*)

(MRSA: methicillin-resistant *Staphylococcus aureus*)

microorganisms, all but few patients present with sepsis with hemodynamic instability. Accordingly, the patient may have to be resuscitated and managed in a high-dependency unit or intensive care unit with intravenous fluids, inotropes, and occasionally specific medications such as albumin or intravenous immunoglobulin (IVIG) in streptococcal TSS. A recent meta-analysis suggests that mortality (both 30-day and 90-day) is significantly reduced in the patients who have received a combination of clindamycin and IVIG. On the contrary, the results from a recent systematic review on the benefits of hyperbaric oxygen therapy in the management of NF have been equivocal.

Prevention

Virulent strains of GAS from a patient affected with NF may spread by droplet infection in close contacts which may cause the illness rarely. Thus, the contacts should be educated about prevention and seeking early medical help if symptoms develop.

NECROTIZING FASCIITIS AFFECTING SPECIFIC REGIONS

Perineum (Fournier Gangrene)

Necrotizing fasciitis of the perineum is a polymicrobial infection that occurs due to a breach in the gastrointestinal or urethral mucosa. Common among the patients with diabetes mellitus, the syndrome is abrupt in onset with severe pain that may spread rapidly to other adjoining areas such as the anterior abdominal wall and the gluteal muscles. It is more common in men with the involvement of the scrotum and penis, while it may involve the labia in women.[4]

Head and Neck

Any breach in the mucosa of the upper aerodigestive tract due to surgery, instrumentation, or spontaneous infection can cause NF of the head and neck. Often polymicrobial infection includes both aerobes and anaerobes, most are attributable to dental etiology. The spread can be rapid to involve the face, lower neck, or even the mediastinum. If not treated promptly, NF in the neck can lead to airway compromise or jugular vein suppurative thrombosis (Lemierre syndrome).

PROGNOSIS

Despite the best possible therapy, NF in adults is associated with significant mortality in the range of 14–40%, particularly the Fournier gangrene and monomicrobial NF. The mortality may be due to several general and specific factors (**Box 6**).

> **BOX 6: Factors associated with increased mortality in necrotizing fasciitis (NF).**
>
> *General factors:*
> - Age >60 years
> - White blood cell count >30,000/L^{-3}; band forms >10%
> - Serum creatinine >2.0 mg/dL
> - Delay in surgery >24 hours
>
> *Specific factors:*
> - NF involving the head, neck, thorax, or abdomen
> - Streptococcal toxic shock syndrome (TSS)
> - Clostridial infection

REFERENCES

1. Tan JH, Koh BT, Hong CC, Lim SH, Liang S, Chan GWH, et al. A comparison of necrotising fasciitis in diabetics and non-diabetics: a review of 127 patients. Bone Joint J. 2016;98-B(11):1563-68.
2. Cheng NC, Tai HC, Chang SC, Chang CH, Lai HS. Necrotizing fasciitis in patients with diabetes mellitus: clinical characteristics and risk factors for mortality. BMC Infect Dis. 2015;15:417.
3. Khamnuan P, Chongruksut W, Jearwattanakanok K, Patumanond J, Tantraworasin A. Necrotizing fasciitis: epidemiology and clinical predictors for amputation. Int J Gen Med. 2015;8:195-202.
4. Zhang Z, Liu P, Yang B, Li J, Wang W, Yang H, et al. Necrotizing fasciitis caused by diabetic foot. Int J Infect Dis. 2021;103:3-5.

CHAPTER 13

VS RAMACHANDRAN

Vilayanur Subramanian Ramachandran is an Indian-American neuroscientist, known for his experiments and theories in behavioral neurology and the invention of the mirror box which has an important role in the management of the phantom limb pain, after amputation. He completed his medical education from Stanley Medical College, India, and went on to obtain his PhD from the University of Cambridge. He invented mirror therapy to treat phantom limb pain and restore motor therapy in weakened limbs of stroke victims. Despite its introduction in the 1990s, most research on its use has been published only after 2009. Dr Ramachandran is the author of many popular books in neurology and has given various talks and lectures. He is also the recipient of various honors, including the Henry Dale Medal and the Padma Bhushan.

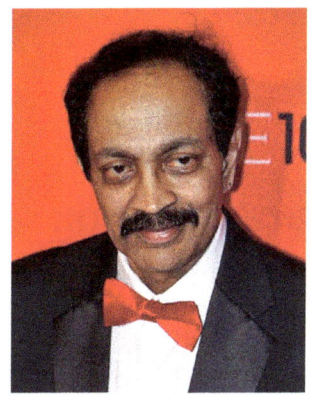

Recent Advances in Diabetic Foot Management

Sandeep Kumar Agarwal, Felix Jebasingh K, Nihal Thomas

INTRODUCTION

Diabetic foot ulcers (DFUs) are a critical complication of diabetes mellitus that induces a significant level of morbidity, mortality, and escalates healthcare costs. Up to one-fifth of patients tend to have DFUs in their lifetime and nearly 85% of them end up having some form of lower limb amputation.[1,2] In this chapter, we discuss the recent updates regarding adjuvant agents that had evidence in improving the outcomes in patients with DFU.

THERMAL MONITORING FOR PREVENTION OF DIABETIC FOOT ULCER

Regular measurement of foot temperature may help in predicting DFUs, thereby reducing their engagement in physical activity thereby further reducing the likelihood of developing a future DFU (**Fig. 1**).

ELIMINATING THE CHALLENGES IN OFFLOADING

The key aspects of successful offloading include:
- Achieving optimal pressure relief with the available offloading
- Monitoring the dosing of activity and physical stress
- Thermal monitoring to detect the preulcerative stage in DFU
- Ensuring compliance and adherence toward offloading devices[3]

There are monitoring offloading and communicating devices that may be inserted as an insole available to assess the pressure values across the foot which thereby help in limiting the pressure and preventing the foot ulcers. However, the major limitation in sensor-based technology is the need for regular calibration of the sensors. There is abundant ongoing research across the globe toward developing low-cost sensors.

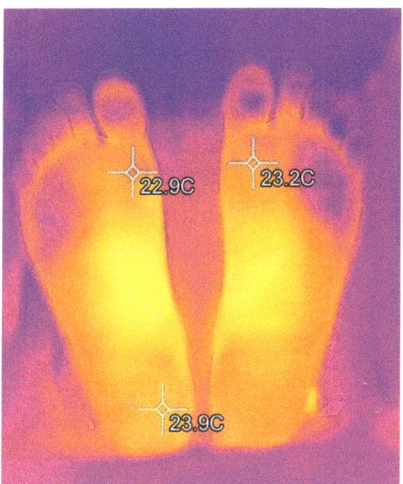

FIG. 1: Infrared camera image using forward-looking infrared (FLIR) one infrared camera.

More recently, technology has helped in optimizing the offloading capacity of devices, in providing feedback regarding physical activity profiles, and in monitoring tissue health with thermometry.

The following are the various areas of research on treatment aspects that were developed in the therapy for DFU (**Table 1**).

Of the therapies discussed in **Table 1**, Manuka honey and larval therapy with bottle green flies have been shown to possess antibacterial effects that were found to be beneficial compared to the standard dressings. However, Manuka honey and larval therapy in an aseptic environment are expensive.

Hyperbaric oxygen therapy (HBOT) offers 100% oxygen and had also shown promising improvement in decreasing the duration of the wound healing; however, they lack large scale randomized controlled studies.

Nutritional Supplements

Nutritional supplements with zinc sulfate, cholecalciferol, and omega-3 fatty acids have been found to be beneficial but lack long-term placebo-controlled studies.

Silver Dressings

Silver ions are known to have antibiotic properties. Hence, dressings composed of grid structure sodium carboxymethyl cellulose and a 1.2% silver ion has broad-spectrum antibacterial properties. The sliver impregnated dressings release the silver ions continuously and slowly that induces a negative charge on the bacterial cell membrane which prevents them from further replication of the bacteria. Moreover, it causes generation of a moist environment over the ulcer surface leading to granulation, angiogenesis, and rapid migration of epidermal cells. Silver

TABLE 1: Efficacy of adjuvant therapies in diabetic foot ulcer (DFU) therapy.[4-7]

Therapies tried	Wound healing benefit versus standard of care
Nonsurgical debridement	
Hydrogels	No clear benefit in decreasing the number of days in wound healing
Clostridial collagenase ointment	No clear benefit
Maggot/larval therapy	There are few studies which have shown benefits in a controlled setting
Hydrosurgery	No apparent benefit
Dressings and topical agents	
Honey	Manuka honey has shown benefit in reducing the rate of amputations in patients with DFU
Other topical antimicrobials	Unclear benefit
Oxygen therapies	
Topical oxygen	Increasing evidence of its efficacy in both RCTs and meta-analyses[8]
Hyperbaric oxygen therapy	No apparent benefit in long-term healing
Acellular bioproducts	
Acellular bioproducts	Has shown benefit in few studies. However, these studies have bias in choosing patients
Human growth factors	
Fibroblast growth factor	Unclear benefit
Epidermal growth factor	Unclear benefit
Vascular endothelial growth factor	Apparent benefit, but limited data
Granulocyte colony-stimulating factor	No apparent benefit
Platelet-derived growth factor	Apparent benefit in small sample-sized studies
Skin graft and bioengineered skin	
Skin graft and bioengineered skin	Apparent benefit, but randomized controlled studies had observers' bias
Energy-based therapies	
Electrical stimulation	No beneficial effects
Shockwave therapy	No beneficial effects
Electromagnetic therapy	No beneficial effects
Laser therapy	No beneficial effects
Phototherapy	No beneficial effects
Miscellaneous therapies	
Stem cell therapy	Few anecdotal case reports. Otherwise lacks large scale studies

impregnated therapies are found to be effective though there appears to be limited data to support their use.

TOPICAL OXYGEN THERAPY

Oxygen (O_2) can facilitate the process of wound repair as it is an essential co-factor for oxygen-dependent enzymes that are crucial for the process of wound healing. Topical oxygen therapy (TOT) has been used for clinical purposes for several decades.

Topical oxygen therapy delivery is achieved through three general types of delivery, which can be both ambulatory and home-based. These include: (1) continuous delivery of oxygen (CDO) at negligible pressures, (2) low constant pressure delivery in a contained chamber, and (3) higher cyclically pressurized and humidified delivery in a contained extremity chamber.

The latest systematic reviews with meta-analyses have pointed out the clinical effectiveness of TOT for healing chronic diabetic foot ulcers (DFUs). It has also been indicated that TOT (using cyclically pressurized devices and CDO) significantly improves wound healing in chronic DFUs. Resulting from the increasing evidence to support the use of TOT for treating chronic DFUs, TOT prescription guidelines have been established through a Delphi consensus by an expert, multidisciplinary panel.[8,9]

TOPICAL SUCROSE OCTASULFATE—IMPREGNATED DRESSINGS (URGOSTART) AND TOPICAL FIBRIN AND LEUKOCYTE PLATELET PATCH (LEUCOPATCH)

Expression of matrix metalloproteinases (MMPs) can be exaggerated in chronic wounds, which can lead to abnormal tissue breakdown and increased healing duration. Incorporation of sucrose octasulfate (UrgoStart) into a nonadherent, novel form of dressing can impede the action of MMPs.

A recent multicenter, double-blinded randomized controlled trial (RCT) reported statistically significant benefit in healing time from the usage of this dressing, when compared to a placebo. The United Kingdom National Institute for Care and Clinical Excellence has also approved the product for use in neuropathic ulcers.[10,11]

Another option for treating nonhealing ulcers is the use of platelet-rich plasma or fibrin, which might promote healing of DFUs by supporting release of growth factors and cytokines responsible for angiogenesis, and tissue repair.

Multilayered patches consisting of autologous leukocytes (LeucoPatch), fibrin, and platelets have been developed recently. These can be produced at the bedside, without the addition of any reagents. Use of such patches was evaluated in another large, multicenter, multinational, outcome-blinded RCT for patients with hard-to-heal ulcers, palpable foot pulses, or ankle-brachial index (ABI) of the index limb ≥0.7. Overall, the study found that complete healing was achieved in significantly more ulcers by 20 weeks in the intervention group than in the group receiving standard of care. However, the International Working Group on the Diabetic Foot (IWGDF) guidelines indicate a cautious recommendation for using this intervention considering limited evidence and lower cost-effectiveness.[12,13]

Three-dimensional Printing and Insoles for Footwear

Three-dimensional (3D) printed insoles help to improve the foot health of patients with diabetes, especially in patients with Charcot foot, wherein arches of foot are altered.

CONCLUSION

The standard strategies that are followed to manage DFU are wound debridement, dressings to maintain moist wound setting and to control exudate, offloading a wound, assessment of the vessels, to control infection, ischemia, and hyperglycemia management.

All these are best followed at the hospital setting with multiple disciplines to manage DFUs. Key aspects of successful offloading diabetic feet is achieving optimal offloading, adherence with offloading devices, and optimizing the user experience.

REFERENCES

1. Armstrong DG, Boulton AJM, Bus SA. Diabetic foot ulcers and their recurrence. New Engl J Med. 2017;376(24):2367-75.
2. Walsh JW, Hoffstad OJ, Sullivan MO, Margolis DJ. Association of diabetic foot ulcer and death in a population-based cohort from the United Kingdom. Diabet Med. 2016;33(11):1493-8.
3. Hinchliffe RJ, Forsythe RO, Apelqvist J, Boyko EJ, Fitridge R, Hong JP, et al. Guidelines on diagnosis, prognosis, and management of peripheral artery disease in patients with foot ulcers and diabetes (IWGDF 2019 update). Diabetes Metab Res Rev. 2020;36 Suppl 1:e3276.
4. Everett E, Mathioudakis N. Update on management of diabetic foot ulcers. Ann NY Acad Sci. 2018;1411(1):153-65.
5. Elraiyah T, Pablo Domecq J, Prutsky G, Tsapas A, Nabhan M, Frykberg RG. A systematic review and meta-analysis of débridement methods for chronic diabetic foot ulcers. 2016;63(2s):37s-47s.
6. Crews RT, Yalla SV, Dhatt N, Burdi D, Hwang S. Monitoring location-specific physical activity via integration of accelerometry and geotechnology within patients with or at risk of diabetic foot ulcers: a technological report. J Diabetes Sci Technol. 2017;11(5):899-903.
7. Kasiewicz LN, Whitehead KA. Recent advances in biomaterials for the treatment of diabetic foot ulcers. Biomater Sci. 2017;5(10):1962-75.
8. Frykberg RG, Franks PJ, Edmonds M, Brantley JN, Teot L, Wild R, et al. A Multinational, Multicenter, Randomized, Double-Blinded, Placebo-Controlled Trial to Evaluate the Efficacy of Cyclical Topical Wound Oxygen (TWO2) therapy in the treatment of chronic diabetic foot ulcers: The TWO2 study. Diabetes Care. 2020;43(3):616-24.
9. Boulton AJM, Armstrong DG, Londahl M, Frykberg RG, Game FL, Edmonds ME, et al. New Evidence-Based Therapies for Complex Diabetic Foot Wounds. Arlington (VA): American Diabetes Association; 2022.
10. Edmonds M, Lázaro-Martínez JL, Alfayate-Garcia JM, Martini J, Petit JM, Rayman G, et al. Sucrose octasulfate dressing versus control dressing in patients with neuroischaemic diabetic foot ulcers (Explorer): an international, multicentre, double-blind, randomised, controlled trial. Lancet Diabetes Endocrinol. 2018;6:186-96.
11. National Institute for Health and Care Excellence. UrgoStart for treating diabetic foot ulcers and leg ulcers. [online] Available from https://www.nice.org.uk/guidance/mtg42/resources/urgostart-for-treating-diabetic-foot-ulcers-and-leg-ulcers-pdf-64372052418757. [Last accessed July, 2022].
12. Game F, Jeffcoate W, Tarnow L, Jacobsen JL, Whitham DJ, Harrison EF, et al. LeucoPatch system for the management of hard-to-heal diabetic foot ulcers in the UK, Denmark, and Sweden: an observer-masked, randomised controlled trial. Lancet Diabetes Endocrinol. 2018;6:870-8.
13. Rayman G, Vas P, Dhatariya K, Driver V, Hartemann A, Londahl M, et al. Guidelines on use of interventions to enhance healing of chronic foot ulcers in diabetes (IWGDF 2019 update). Diabetes Metab Res Rev. 2020;36(Suppl. 1):e3283.

INDEX

Page numbers followed by *b* refer to box, *f* refer to figure, *fc* refer to flowchart, and *t* refer to table.

A

Abduction 16
Above-knee amputation 167
Abscess 160
Achilles
  tendon, shortening of 30
  tenotomy 166
Adduction 16
Adjuvant therapy, efficacy of 182*t*
Advanced glycation end-products 27
Aeromonas hydrophila 170
Air cast boot 83*f*
Alcohol consumption, chronic 29
Aldose reductase inhibitor 41
Allodynia 29
Alpha-lipoic acid 40
Amitriptyline 38
Amoxicillin 59
Amputation 151, 162, 166
  partial 167
  previous 161
  type of 167
Amyloidosis 29
Amyotrophy 26
Angiogram 105
Angioplasty 166
Angle-closure glaucoma 38
Ankle 9, 69, 71
  and foot complex, motions of 16
  brachial pressure index 52, 105, 106*f*, 107, 108, 111, 114
  foot orthosis 62, 82*f*, 125
    patellar tendon-bearing 127
  joint 14, 66*f*
  nerve supply of 15*f*
  pressure 108
  varus deformity of 127*f*
Anorexia 172
Antibiotic 165
  carbapenem group of 176
  duration of 100, 101, 165

resistance 165
therapy 163, 164, 176
  duration of 101*t*
toxicity 165
Antiphospholipid antibodies 28
Arsenic 29
Arteriovenous systems 3
Artery
  anterior tibial 15
  bypass graft, postcoronary 121
Arthrodesis 166
Arthropathy
  active 78
  inactive 78
Articulations 11
Asymmetric lower limb motor
  neuropathy 26
Autonomic dysfunction 3
Autonomic neuropathy 19, 26, 140

B

Below-knee amputation 115*f*, 167
Bilateral great toe dorsal foot ulcers 143*f*
Biopsy 81
Biothesiometer 35*f*
Blood
  glucose 24
    management 42
    rapid correction of 29
  sugars 128
  urea nitrogen 36
Bohler iron cast 61*f*, 121, 122, 122*f*, 123*f*
Bone 10
  biopsy 81, 98
  fusion of 87
  involvement 55, 60
  marrow
    abnormality, location of 79
    edema 72*f*, 77*f*, 84, 85
  necrosis 165
  scan 80, 80*f*

Index

Bony prominence, excision of 87
Brachial blood pressure index 52
Brodsky's anatomic-based classification systems 71
Burns 151

C

Calcaneal periosteum 97*f*
Calcaneal pitch 74, 75*f*, 76*f*, 87
Calcaneocuboid-intertarsal joint 69
Calcaneovalgus 22*f*
Calcaneovarus 22*f*
Calcium channel modulators 38
Callosities 138
Callus removal 57, 135
Capsaicin 39
Carbapenem 176
 therapy 164
Cardiovascular disease 27
Cefotaxime 176
Ceftriaxone 59, 176
Cellulitis 50*t*, 51*f*, 85, 160
Cephalexin 59
Cephalosporins 176
Charcot's arthropathy 69, 70, 125, 126*f*, 128
 classification for 71
 diabetes-related 3
Charcot's foot 3, 52*f*, 66, 73, 77-80, 84, 85, 87, 98, 98*t*, 123, 125
 active 72*f*, 77*f*
 acute 73*f*, 76*f*, 77*f*, 79
 chronic 70*f*, 72*f*-76*f*, 78*f*, 86, 87
 diagnosis of early-stage 76
 management of 81, 86
 middle- to late-stage 77
 offloading of 82*f*
Charcot's joints 70
Charcot's neuroarthropathy 30, 73
 exostectomy of 166
Charcot's neuropathic osteoarthropathy 3
Charcot's neuropathy 5
Charcot's restraint orthotic walker 62, 82
Charcot's walker 83*f*
Cilastatin 60
Ciprofloxacin 60
Claudication pain 30
Claustrophobia 80
Clavulanate 59
Claw toe 52*f*

Clindamycin 59, 60, 176
Clostridial collagenase ointment 182
Clostridial infection 178
Collagen sponge 164
Color Doppler ultrasound 105
Computed tomography 99
 angiogram 105, 107, 114
 scan 79, 80
Contrast-enhanced computed tomography scan 173
Contrast-enhanced magnetic resonance angiogram 105, 107
Corneal confocal microscopy 35
Coronary artery disease 121
Cortical fractures 77
Cranial mononeuropathy 31
Cranial nerve 31
Cranial neuropathy 26, 31
C-reactive protein 73, 94, 173
Creatinine 173
Crepitus 162, 172
Cuboid
 forming lowermost bone 72*f*
 fragmentation of 73*f*
 height 74

D

Daptomycin 176
Debridement 56, 162
 extent of 165
Deep fascia 12
Deep peroneal nerve 14
Deformity 6
Depressed tendon reflexes 29
Desipramine 38
Devitalized tissues, debridement of 161
Diabetes Control and Complications Trial 40
Diabetes mellitus 2, 24, 27*f*, 44, 69, 110*f*, 111*f*, 113*f*, 135, 160, 169, 171
 type 1 25, 70
 type 2 24, 70, 90, 119, 121, 125, 128, 130, 131, 150
Diabetic amyotrophy 41
 treatment of 41
Diabetic foot 2, 3, 9, 34*f*, 51, 118, 119*t*
 anatomy of 9
 assessment of risk of 6*f*
 biomechanics of 9

Index

care 2
complications 44
disease 2, 118, 160
fissures in 140
infection 160, 164
   severity of 55t, 59t
   surgical treatment of 161b
   types of 160b
management 180
osteomyelitis 90, 91, 96b, 100b, 160, 163b, 167t
   antibiotic treatment of 164
   diagnosis of 99t
   pathogenesis of 91
surgeries in 160
therapy 144f
ulcer 2, 44, 46, 58, 104, 151, 157, 160, 162b, 180
   classification of 46, 95t
   etiology of 46
   infection in 163t
   pathogenesis of 46fc
   prevalence of 135, 180
   therapy 182t
Diabetic neuropathy 2, 19, 25, 36fc, 42
Diabetic retinopathy 44
Diabetic sensorimotor polyneuropathy 41
Diarrhea 172
Diffuse bone marrow edema 72f
Digital subtraction angiogram 105, 114
Distal trans tibiofibular amputation 167
Doppler arterial flow studies 52
Dorsalis pedis 123
Dorsiflexion 16
Doxycycline 59, 176
Duloxetine 38
Dundee classification 50t
  modified 50

E

Ecchymosis 172
Eichenholtz classification system 71
Electrical spinal cord stimulation 40, 42
Electromagnetic nerve stimulation, frequency-modulated 40
Electromagnetic therapy 182
Electromyography 29
  nerve conduction velocity 35
Entrapment neuropathy 31

Epidermal growth factor 182
Epithelial edge advancement 57
Equinus deformity 129f
Ertapenem 60
Erythema 51, 172
Erythrocyte sedimentation rate 73, 94
Escherichia coli 91, 170
Exostectomy 87, 166
Extensive necrosis 162

F

Fabry's disease 29
Fasciitis 169
Fasciotomy 162
Femoral neuropathy 31
Fever 172
Fiber
  diameter velocity 26
  neuropathy, large 29, 37
Fibroblast growth factor 182
Fibula 11
Fissures 140, 145f
  over bilateral hind foot 141f
Flat foot 14
Flexor digitorum
  brevis 12
  longus 11
Flexor hallucis
  brevis 12
  longus 11
Fluorodeoxyglucose 80
Folic acid 41
Foot 66, 78
  amputations, levels of 167f
  arches of 13, 14f
  blood supply of 15f
  bones of 10f
  care 135, 145
  clinical image of 68f
  complex 9
  extrinsic muscles of 11
  functional segments of 11f
  infection 114, 160
    classification 108f
  internal structure of sole of 12
  muscles of 47f
  nerve supply of 15f
  perfusion, restoration of 111
  plantar aspect of 145f

Index

ulcer 19, 21, 25, 45f, 51, 133, 140
   classification of 53, 54t
   depth of 93
   management of 53, 144
   recurrent 50
   width of 93
   X-ray of 73
Forefoot 55
   bones of 11
   joint of 11
Fournier gangrene 169, 177
Fractures, acute neuropathic 86
Fungal nail 145f

G

Gabapentin 38
Gait 18, 37
   cycle 18, 18f
Gamma aminobutyric acid 38
Gangrene 55, 162
Gastrocnemius 11
Gastrointestinal tract 25
Genitourinary tract 25
Ghost sign 79
Glucose 173
Glycemic control 40, 165
Gouty arthritis 85
Granulocyte colony-stimulating
   factor 182

H

Hallux valgus 129, 136
Hammer toes 30
Heart
   disease, ischemic 128
   rate 50
Heavy metal poisoning 29
Heel strike 18
Hemoglobin 5, 173
Hemostasis 161
Hindfoot 10, 11, 91
   Charcot deformity 166t
   forefoot angle 74
   joint of 11
   ulcer 93f
Hospital infection control
   committee 164, 176
Human immunodeficiency virus
   infection 29

Hydrogels 182
Hydrosurgery 182
Hyperalgesia 29
Hyperbaric oxygen therapy 181, 182
Hyperglycemia 5, 27
Hyperkeratosis 136
Hyperpigmentation 124f
Hypotension 172

I

Imipramine 38
Immune hypothesis 28
Immunoglobulin, intravenous 177
Immunosuppression 171
Impenem 60
Infection
   acute 164
   bacterial 56
   grade of 163
   mild 164
   moderate 164
   severe 164
   treatment of 119
Infectious Disease Society of America 99
Inflammatory demyelinating
   polyneuropathy, chronic 36
Insulin
   like growth factor 28
   neuritis 29
International Working Group of
   Diabetic Foot 34, 50, 108, 118
Interphalangeal joint 69, 71
Intertarsal joints 77f
Intrinsic muscles 12
Irrigation 161
Ischemia 108, 114, 162

J

Joint 11
   axis 16f
   destruction 77
   dislocations 77
   effusion 78f
   mobility 19, 20

L

Large-fiber neuropathies 28fc
Larval therapy 182

Index

Laser therapy 182
Leg, severe ischemia of 109
Levofloxacin 59, 60
Life-threatening sepsis 162, 166
Limb ischemia 165
Limb-threatening infections 166
Linezolid 60
Lipoprotein, low high-density 27
Liver 24
Local wound care 119
Longitudinal arch, medial 14
Lower leg, bones of 11

M

Macrostrain 152
Macular edema 24
Maggot therapy 182
Malaise 172
Marine-water infection 176*b*
Meary's angle 73, 74*f*, 76*f*, 82
Mechanical offloading 81
Medical management 81
Medical therapy 109
　failure of 165
　primarily 165
　role of 165*t*
Meleney ulcer 169
Metabolic control 119
Metabolic hypothesis 27
Metatarsal fracture 85
Metatarsophalangeal joint 21, 69, 71, 73*f*, 77*f*, 86
　dislocation of 76*f*
　proximal 92*f*
Methicillin-resistant *Staphylococcus aureus* 58, 164, 169, 176
Methylene diphosphonate 99
Microalbuminuria 44
Microbiological control 58
Microcellular rubber 37
Microcirculatory disturbances 105
Microstrain 152
Microvascular hypothesis 28
Microvascular insufficiency 28
Midfoot 10, 55, 91
　acute charcot 86
　bones of 11
　joint of 11
　ulcer 94*f*, 124*f*

Minimal bone marrow edema 78*f*
Moisture balance 57
Monoclonal gammopathy 31
Monofilament 32*b*
　method of 33
　testing 32
　types of 32*f*
Mononeuritis multiplex 26
Mononeuropathy 31
Morton's neuroma 30
Motion, ankle joint range of 17*f*
Motor neuropathy 3, 19, 26
Moxifloxacin 59
Multidisciplinary team 135
Multiple myeloma 29
Muscles 11
Myalgias 172
Myelination 25*f*
Myositis 169

N

Nail care 146
Naviculocuneiform joint 69
Necrotizing adipositis 169
Necrotizing fasciitis 162, 169, 170, 170*t*, 172*b*, 173*t*, 176, 176*b*, 177, 178*b*
　clinical features in 172*t*
　intraoperative features of 174*b*
　pathological features of 174*b*
　risk factors for 171*b*
　surgical options in 174*t*
Necrotizing soft-tissue infection 160, 169, 172*f*, 175*f*
Negative pressure wound therapy 56, 150, 152, 153, 157, 157*f*, 166
Nerve
　biopsy 35
　classification 26
　conduction
　　study 35, 41
　　velocity 26, 36
　growth factor 28
　ischemia of 31
　supply 14
Neuroischemic ulcer 48
　over great toe 49*f*
Neurologic impairment score 36
Neurologic symptoms score 36
Neuropathic ulcer 46, 47*f*, 49*t*

Index

Neuropathy 19, 35, 46, 56, 161
  acute painful 29
  asymmetric 31
  chronic painful 29
  diffuse 28
  medical therapy for 42
Neurotrophic factors, deficiency of 28
Neurotrophic hypothesis 28
Neutrophilic leukocytosis 44
Newer techniques 35
Non-invasive tests 105
Non-neuropathic fractures 86
Nonproliferative diabetic retinopathy 24
Nonsteroidal anti-inflammatory drugs 31, 38, 171
Normocytic anemia 44
Nortriptyline 38
Nuclear medicine imaging 80
Nutritional supplements 181

O

Obesity 171
Opioids 39
Optimal antibiotic therapy 165
Osteoarthritis 30
Osteoarthropathy 161
Osteomyelitis 73f, 79, 80, 85, 91, 92, 92f, 93f, 98, 98t, 160
  chronic 96f
  diagnosis of 98
  microbiology of 91
  predictive of 93
Osteopenia 127f
Oxycodone 39
Oxygen saturation 50

P

Pacemaker 80
Pain 51
  severe 66, 172
Painful diabetic neuropathy 37
  peripheral 30t
  treatment of 37, 40
Pamidronate 81
Paronychia 160
Patellar tendon bearing 62, 127
  orthosis 128f
Pedal pulses intact 55
Penicillin 176

Peptide, calcitonin gene-related 69
Percutaneous electrical nerve stimulation 42
Percutaneous femoral angioplasty 113f
Perfusion extent depth infection sensation 163
Perineum 169, 177
Peripheral arterial disease 2, 4fc, 5, 6, 52, 104, 106f, 107, 114fc, 115, 161, 171
Peripheral nerves
  classification of 25f
  system 25
Peripheral neuropathy 3, 19, 24, 25, 41, 44, 69, 150, 161
  diabetes-related 27
  pathogenesis of 27
  risk factors for 27
Peripheral sensory neuropathy 25
Peripheral vascular disease 19, 46, 104
Peroneal artery 15
Persistent soft tissue 165
Pes planus 14
Phalanges 10, 11
Phalanx 10
Photo plethysmography 106
Photoplethysmogram 105
Photoplethysmography 52
Phototherapy 182
Piperacillin 60, 176
Plantar aponeurosis 18
Plantar fascia 12, 12f
Plantar fasciitis 30
Plantar flexion 16
  deformity correction 166
Plantar tissue thickness 21
Plaster of Paris 122
Platelet-derived growth factor 182
Podiatric procedures 166
Polyneuropathy, chronic inflammatory demyelinating 31
Positron emission tomography 80
Post-transmetatarsal amputation 45f
Pregnancy 171
Pressure
  magnitude of 20
  reduces 57
  relief of 119
  repetition of 20
  sores 151
Probe-to-bone test 93
  positive 49

Index

Procalcitonin 94
Protective sensation, loss of 4, 6, 32, 33, 50
Protein gene product 35
Pseudomonas aeruginosa 59, 91
Pulse
  palpable 55
  volume recording 106
  wave recording waveforms 105, 107

Q

Quantitative autonomic function tests 36
Quantitative sensory tests 26, 36

R

Radiculopathy 30
Radionuclide scanning 98
Randomized controlled trial 38, 157
Ray amputation 167
Recent surgery 171
Reconstructive surgery 165
Rehabilitation 135
Renal failure 161
Renal insufficiency 50
Respiratory rate 50
Rocker foot deformity 72*f*

S

Salicylic acid 141*f*, 142*f*
Sanders and Frykberg classification 71, 72*f*, 83, 84, 86, 87
Saphenous nerve 14
Sclerosis 73*f*
Scrotum 169
Sensorimotor polyneuropathy 26
Sensory ataxia 30
Sensory modalities 26
Sensory nerve fibers 25
  types of 26, 26*t*
Sensory neuropathy 19, 162
Septic arthritis 160
Serotonin norepinephrine reuptake inhibitors 38
Serotonin reuptake inhibitors 38
Serum inflammatory markers 94
Sesamoid bones 10, 11
Shockwave therapy 182
Silicone bunion shield 129
Silver dressings 181
Sinbad classification 55*t*

Single-photon emission computed tomography 99
Sinus tracts 79
Skin 12
  blebs 172
  graft 182
    failed 151
  perfusion
    pressure 105, 107
    restoration of 119
  ulceration 79
Sloughy tissue 57
Small-fiber
  neuropathy 28*fc*, 37
  polyneuropathy 26
Sodium 173
Sodium-channel blockers 39
Soft tissue 21, 60
  infections 169
    classification of 169*t*
Staphylococcus
  aureus 59, 91
  epidermidis 91
Stasis ulcers 151
Stem cell therapy 182
Streptococcal toxic shock syndrome 178
Streptococcus species 59
Subchondral cysts 78*f*, 79
Subclinical neuropathy 26
Subcutaneous fat 79
Subtalar joint 17*f*, 69, 71
Subungual ulcer 58*f*
Sudomotor function devices 35
Sulfamethoxa 59
Sulfamethoxazole 176
Superficial fascia 12, 13
Superficial peroneal nerve 14
Sural nerve 14
Surgery 109
Surgical debridement 162, 176
Surgical management 161
Surgical preventive strategies 166
Surgical sharp debridement 57
Swelling 67
Syme amputation 133
Syme prosthesis 133
Systemic inflammation 164
Systemic inflammatory response syndrome 163
Systolic blood pressure 50

T

Tabes dorsalis 69
Tachycardia 172
Talus 10, 11
Tarsal joints 71
Tarsal tunnel syndrome 30
Tarsometatarsal amputation 167
Tarsometatarsal joint 69, 71, 77*f*, 83, 84
   destruction of 127*f*
Tazobactam 60, 176
Technetium-99m methylene diphosphonate 80
Tendo-Achilles 129
Tendons 11
Therapeutic intent, surgical management with 161
Thyroid function tests 24
Thyroid-stimulating hormone 36
Tibia 11
   dry skin over shin of 145*f*
Tibial angioplasty 113*f*
Tibial artery, posterior 15
Tibial nerve, posterior 14
Tibialis posterior 11
Tissue debridement 57
Toe
   amputation 167
   brachial index 105, 106*f*, 107, 114
   pressure 105, 106*f*, 108
Topical agents 39
Topical oxygen 182
Total contact cast 61*f*, 62, 81, 86, 121
   role of 81
Total negative pressure technology 151
Toxic shock syndrome 171
Tramadol 39
Transcutaneous electrical nerve stimulation 40
Transcutaneous oximetry 52
Transcutaneous oxygen pressure 105, 108
Transmetatarsal amputation 112*f*, 167
   stump ulcer 57*f*
Transverse arch 14
Transverse tarsal amputation 167
Trauma 151, 171
Tricyclic antidepressants 37
Trimethoprim 59, 176
Trophic ulcer 131
Truncal mononeuropathy 26

U

Ulcer 49, 55
   chronic 161
   deep 55, 92*f*
   dressing 53
   following trauma 50
   formation 3
   ischemic 48, 49*t*
   non-healing 118
   protection of 119
   superficial 55

V

Vacuum-assisted closure 151, 155*f*
Vacuum-sealing technique 151
Vancomycin 60, 176
Varus deformity 127*f*, 132*f*
Vascular disease 19
Vascular endothelial growth factor 182
Vibration perception threshold measurement 34
Vibrio vulnificus 170, 176
Vitamin B12 36, 41

W

Waddling gait 30
Wagner–Meggitt classification 55*t*
Walking barefoot 161
Warm foot 30
White blood cell 94, 99, 173
Wifi classification system 108
Windlass mechanism 13
Wound 108, 114
   abdominal 151
   acute 151
   care 165
   chronic 151
   necrotic 164
   open 161
   sternotomy 151
   suction, sealed surface 151

X

X-ray, interpretation of 83

Z

Zoledronic acid 81

EU GSPR Authorised Reprsentative
Logos Europe, 9 rue Nicolas Poussin
1700, La Rochelle, France
Phone: +33 (0) 6 67 93 73 78
E-mail: contact@logoseurope.eu

www.ingramcontent.com/pod-product-compliance
Ingram Content Group UK Ltd.
Pitfield, Milton Keynes, MK11 3LW, UK
UKHW051137270226
468476UK00003B/22